babycare
before
birth

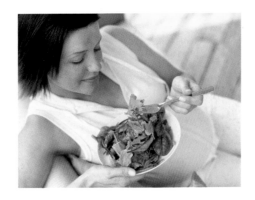

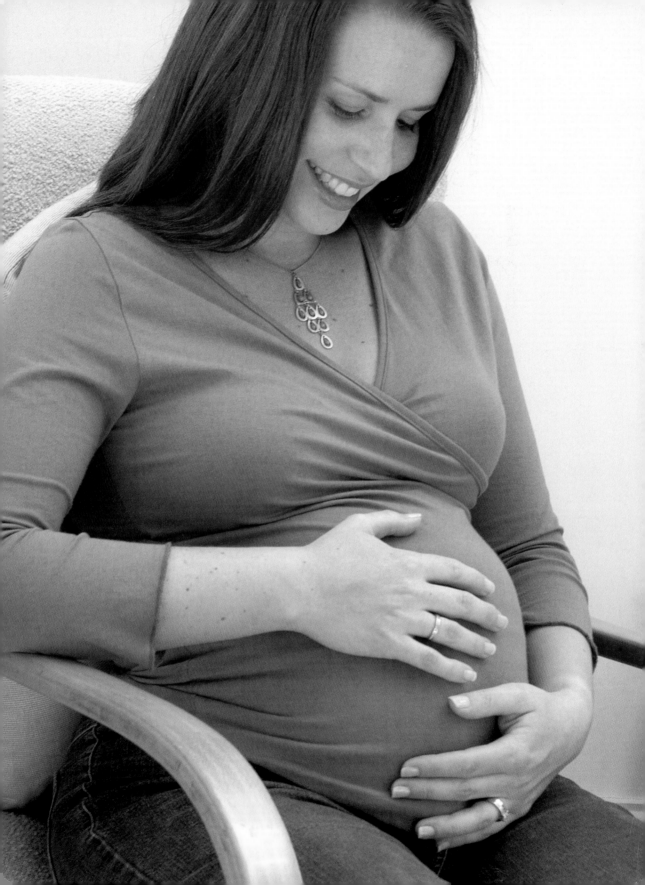

babycare
before
birth

ZITA WEST

Consultant

JOYCE FRYE DO, MBA, FACOG

RESEARCH FELLOW, CENTER FOR CLINICAL EPIDEMIOLOGY AND BIOSTATISTICS,
UNIVERSITY OF PENNSYLVANIA

DK

LONDON, NEW YORK, MUNICH, MELBOURNE, DELHI

Senior editor Esther Ripley
Senior art editor Glenda Fisher
Project editor Angela Baynham
Designer Kathryn Gammon
US senior editor Jill Hamilton
DTP designer Sonia Charbonnier
Production controller Mandy Inness
Managing editor Penny Warren
Managing art editor Marianne Markham
Picture research Bridget Tily
DK picture librarian Romaine Werblow
Jacket designer Neal Cobourne
Jacket editor Adam Powley
Publishing director Corinne Roberts

First published in the United States in 2006 by
DK Publishing, Inc.
375 Hudson Street, New York, NY 10014

A Cataloging-in-Publication record for this book is available from the Library of Congress
ISBN 0-7566-1879-7

DK books are available at special discounts for bulk purchases for sales promotions, premiums, fund-raising, or educational use. For details, contact: DK Publishing Special Markets, 375 Hudson Street, New York, NY 10014 or SpecialSales@dk.com

Reproduced by Colourscan, Singapore
Printed and bound Tien Wah Press in Singapore

See our complete product line at
www.dk.com

contents

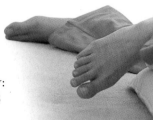

3 Labor, birth, and beyond

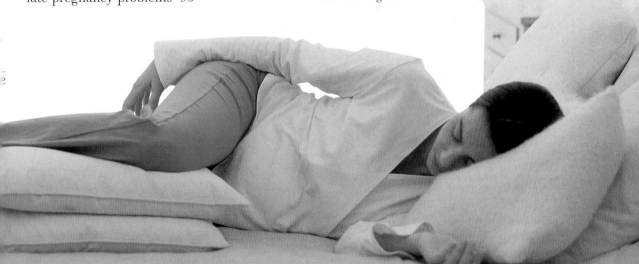

foreword

It was the mid 1990s when, as an obstetrician, I was first introduced to the importance of insuring an adequate intake of DHA for optimizing fetal brain development. (DHA is one of the omega-3 class of Essential Fatty Acids that Zita discusses in the book.) My information source was a prenatal patient who worked as a wholesale representative for a nutritional supplement manufacturer. She had already seen enough research to decide for herself that the risk/benefit ratio was on the side of DHA supplementation, and she had begun taking it. More than 10 years later, an internet search on prenatal DHA got 234,000 hits; yet DHA is not incorporated into most prenatal vitamins, few obstetricians offer substantial dietary advice or recommend it as an additional supplement, and average dietary intake among pregnant women is far lower than standard recommendations.

DHA is just one of the topics that Zita covers in this book that is full of sensible advice and reminders that the best way to

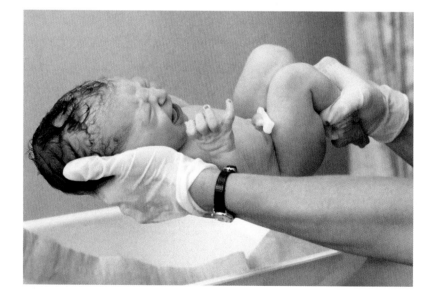

take care of our babies before birth is to take care of ourselves.
For some women, this may require a major shift in priorities
from being focused on career to being focused on motherhood.
The transition can be far greater than first-time mothers
anticipate. By the end of even the easiest of pregnancies, the
burden of swollen feet and carrying an extra 25 pounds forces
some shifting of priorities. (For partners who'd like to
empathize, try strapping on a watermelon and carrying it
24/7 for a while!) Women who go into pregnancy thinking
that they can do it all are often in for some surprises. And
when complications come up, they can go into a tailspin.

The reality is that this is just a taste of what parenting will be
like. I often counseled my patients who were anxious about the
result of one test or another that, as parents, there would
always be worries—they just change as our children move
through developmental stages until we finally worry about
how they are raising our grandchildren. The good news is that
the joy and rewards of parenting are many multiples of the
hours of lost sleep. We cannot be in control of everything, and
the human race is still here; so, in toto, the system works pretty
well. You do the best you can, hope for the best, and then let go
of the rest—no guilt, no "should-haves." This book will help
you do the best you can to take care of yourself and get your
baby off to the healthiest possible start.

JOYCE FRYE DO, MBA, FACOG
Research Fellow, Center for Clinical Epidemiology
and Biostatistics, University of Pennsylvania

author's introduction

Scientists have revealed to us a great deal about fetal development and life in the womb. Even so, I am always amazed that something that starts out as a single cell develops over just nine months into a baby. We are learning more and more, through research and through highly developed scanning techniques, about just how delicate the process is. Research also offers insights into how we can improve the quality of a baby's life while it is still in the uterus—the optimum babycare before birth.

The potential influences on what occurs while your baby is in the uterus are wide ranging and can have an impact throughout its life. Nutritional health has been shown to pass from one generation to the next. For example, the egg from which your life began developed in your mother's ovaries while she was still in your grandmother's womb! When you consider how far back your own nutritional history extends, it becomes clear that the quality of nutrition in your own pregnancy is likely to have an impact on future generations in ways that scientists are only just beginning to understand. A study of women who suffered starvation in Holland at the end of the Second World War, for example, revealed that, although their own daughters were not directly affected, their grandchildren were smaller than average.

Many of the suggestions in the book are based on the work of Professor David Barker, whose research at Southampton University has shown that the growing fetus has incredibly specific peak nutritional requirements at different stages related to the development of its organs and systems. Studies have revealed links between what happens to the fetus in the womb and the development of problems later in life, such as diabetes, high blood pressure, and heart disease. It is now widely believed that childhood allergies and food sensitivities begin in the womb, and that the occurrence of conditions such as preeclampsia and miscarriage can be reduced with the right nutritional approaches. Research has also shown that essential fatty acids, found in certain foods, have a role in brain development in the uterus, and deficiencies can be linked to attention deficit and hyperactivity disorder (ADHD) and learning difficulties in children.

So how can you ensure the best start for your child? I believe in keeping things simple and realistic. I don't expect any woman to put her life on hold for nine months of pregnancy, and you shouldn't feel that you have to. However, I wrote this book because I believe that it is important for you to understand the processes that are going on in your baby's development and respond to them with everyday measures that you can achieve, through diet, stress reduction, and emotional well-being.

I also believe that couples need to prepare to be parents. Ideally, you should be in peak health before conception, which is why my prenatal program begins when you are only thinking about having a baby rather than actually embarking on a pregnancy.

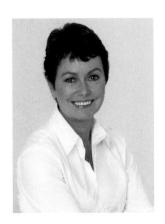

Every pregnancy is different and every woman comes to pregnancy with her unique set of circumstances. But if you adapt the information in this book to suit your needs, you will be doing everything you can to give your baby the best start in life.

Zita West

prenatal program

Your baby's genes are fixed at conception, but you can influence the environment your baby develops in. My prenatal program gives practical recommendations based on scientific research to help you work toward creating a brighter, healthier baby.

GET IT RIGHT FROM THE START

The first chapter of this book focuses on how you prepare yourself for pregnancy. Preconceptual preparation should begin at least three months before you start to try to conceive and is about reviewing your nutrition, fitness, stress levels, and lifestyle in general to see if you relax enough, what your working conditions are like, and whether you take sufficient time off. In particular, nutrition before pregnancy can affect fertility, the early development of the fetus, and a woman's ability to withstand the nutritional demands of pregnancy.

BUILDING NUTRITIONAL FOUNDATIONS

Nutrition throughout pregnancy is a very important part of this book. A developing baby is dependent on its mother's nutritional reserves, some of which will have been built up over weeks, and not on the food she eats on any particular day. The size of the mother's body and her nutrient reserves at the time of conception have an impact on the baby's birthweight. If you are undernourished when you conceive, the amount of food you consume during pregnancy assumes even greater importance. You can "catch up" up to a point, but it is far better to be well nourished from the outset.

Your baby grows as a result of the process of cell division. When nutrition is deficient in the womb, cells divide less frequently, resulting in fewer cells in total in the baby's body, and hence a smaller baby. Your baby will also respond by using its own protein stores for energy.

Undernourishment slows the growth process because of the lack of building blocks, such as proteins, in the diet, and also because of the effect on hormones that control growth, the most important being insulin. If your baby produces less insulin than normal this slows its growth and can have effects into adult life.

Studies have shown that nutritional deficiency while in the womb may lead to disease in later life. If an organ is deprived of key nutrients during early development its growth may be restricted, preventing it from reaching its full potential, and it may not be possible for that organ to restore itself. Building up reserves during the months before you get pregnant will pay dividends and lay great foundations for your pregnancy.

The placenta

This vital organ plays a key role in your baby's development. Difficulties encountered in late pregnancy often originate from how the placenta embedded and developed in early pregnancy. An efficient placenta in the first trimester will ensure a good maternal blood supply, carrying a full range of nutrients to your baby and enabling its organs to develop and grow.

WINDOWS OF OPPORTUNITY

In early development, cells divide and differentiate into specific types of cells with specialist functions. During critical growth "windows," cells are vulnerable to nutrient deficiencies, stress, and exposure to toxins, all of which can affect growth. Within each trimester, you will find "windows of opportunity" features. These will help you to understand how your baby develops and when particular organs are undergoing vital periods of growth. During these windows there may be key nutrients that you can focus on as part of your varied diet, to ensure that a specific organ maximizes its potential for growth and development.

For example, the second trimester is a crucial time for the development of fetal bones. As they start to undergo the process of calcification (hardening) the demand for calcium is high so you need to make sure your diet includes plenty of this important mineral during this trimester (*see* pages 78–9).

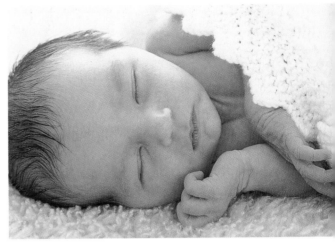

By improving the quality of your baby's life before birth, you can enhance her potential for health after birth and beyond.

LOOKING AT YOUR LIFESTYLE

The way you lead your life can have a major impact on your health during pregnancy as well as the health of your developing baby.

Your baby is constantly monitoring your stress levels by the amount of stress hormones that cross the placenta into the fetal blood supply. The more stress hormones there are in your baby's blood, the more the outside world will appear to be a stressful place. A highly stressful pregnancy will affect the womb environment and mold stress circuits in the fetal brain. These altered stress circuits will affect how your child deals with stress as an adult.

I realize that in modern life there's no escaping stress, but organizing your life in order to minimize it is vitally important. Identify sources of stress, whether they be work, finances or relationships, and then build stress-relieving activities into your day.

As a means of relaxation, stress relief, and taking time out, exercise is of particular importance during pregnancy. Exercise also improves circulation, mobility and flexibility; better muscle tone and stronger joints; raised energy levels; and better posture.

CONNECTING WITH YOUR BABY

Many women worry that they cannot bond with their baby during pregnancy, but spending time focusing on your baby is important, and you can find specific advice on this throughout the book. There is no set formula; we each have our own way of conveying feeling and being receptive. Some of you will be able to close your eyes, relax, and visualize more easily than others. Start by talking to your baby about your hopes and plans, and it will come to recognize your voice. Understanding what a fetus senses and experiences, as well as having an appreciation of its daily rhythms will help you focus better.

We don't often think about the fetus' immediate surroundings, but the womb is its whole world throughout pregnancy. In the warm fluid darkness, supported by your uterine muscle, the fetus is rocked gently by your movements. It constantly receives signals about the outside world that help it learn and practice skills needed to meet challenges beyond the womb. By creating the best possible environment for your pregnancy and your baby, you will send the right messages, so that by the time the baby is born, it will be well along a healthy path of development.

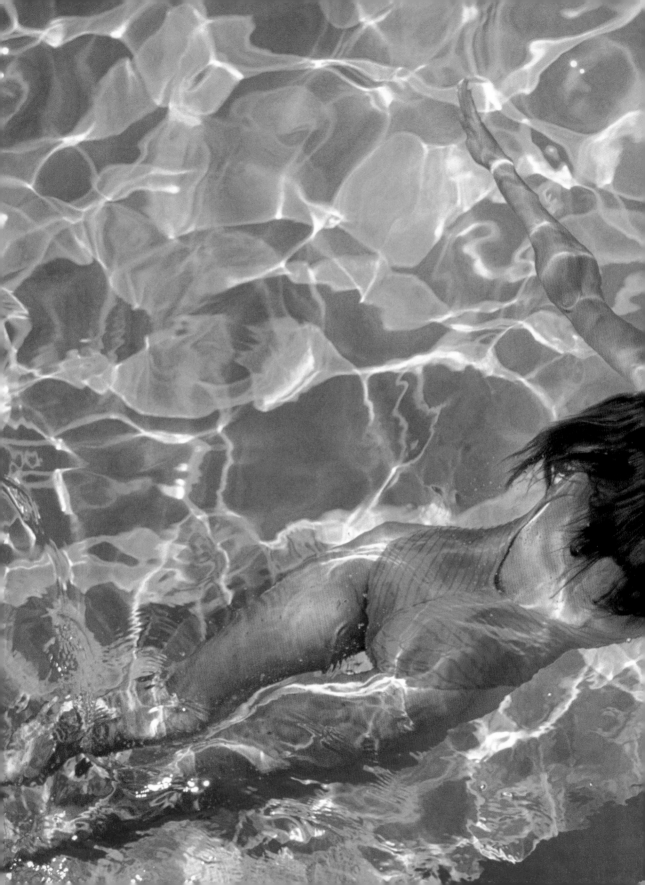

BUILDING BLOCKS

Once you start to consider the possibility of having a baby, it is important to think about the many ways you can prepare, physically, mentally, and emotionally, for the demands of pregnancy and beyond. In this chapter, I take a careful look at the different components of a healthy diet and lifestyle in the buildup to conceiving a baby, as well as the potential impact of modern environmental hazards on fertility. Also included is a section focusing on conception itself and the issues surrounding it.

optimizing fertility

Once you and your partner have decided you want a baby, there are a number of things you need to consider before trying to conceive. You both need to look at the way you live and work toward being as healthy as possible. This is the best way of producing a healthy baby who will grow into a healthy adult.

CHECK YOUR HEALTH

See your gynecologist to discuss your plans and have any necessary tests before you try to conceive.

• Both you and your partner should have a full sexual health screening. Most infections are easily treated but they might cause problems if left.

• Are you immune to rubella? Contracting rubella in early pregnancy can lead to deafness and blindness in the baby.

• Have you had a recent PAP smear? You need to check that there are no precancerous cells in your cervix before you get pregnant.

• If you have any unexplained symptoms, you should be checked for an underlying problem. If you have a disorder such as anemia, asthma, hypertension, thyroid disorders, diabetes, lupus, inflammatory bowel disease, or seizures, you should discuss with your doctor the implications and treatment during conception and pregnancy.

• Both partners should review their family history and ethnic background to see if particular diseases are likely and, if so, undergo genetic screening.

HEALTHY SPERM AND EGGS

Both you and your partner need to prepare in order to produce healthy eggs and sperm. Like all other cells in the body, they need to be able to repair and resist attack from toxins such as free radicals (*see* opposite). Ovaries and testes don't function well if your diet is poor, you use alcohol or drugs, are stressed, or have lots of toxins circulating in your body.

MORE SEX, PLEASE

Many of the couples I see in my conception, fertility, and pregnancy clinic admit to not having sex very often. If you want a baby, it's important to enjoy as much spontaneous passion as possible. The more sex you have, the greater your chance of conceiving.

It's also important to have sex during your fertile period. Ovulation usually occurs between 10 and 16 days before your menstrual period. You are also fertile for up to a week before ovulation, so it's best to get the sperm in position ready for an egg to be released—sperm can survive for two to three days. Pinpointing the exact time of ovulation isn't easy. A predictor kit identifies a surge of luteinizing hormone that occurs about 24 hours before ovulation, but you need to have a good idea of when that will be. If you track your temperature, you will not know until too late that you have ovulated since your temperature rises after ovulation.

You can learn to recognize the telltale signs of fertility: you will feel sexual desire when you are at your most fertile, and your cervical secretions become wetter, clearer, slippery and stretchy, encouraging sperm to swim.

The magnificent egg

An ovum, or egg, is 550 times bigger than a sperm and is the largest cell in the body. Each ovum has a protective outer membrane and structures called mitochondria that produce energy. Inside the ovum's tiny nucleus are the 23 pairs of chromosomes that contain our genetic material, stored in DNA.

Eggs age, as do all body cells, and DNA becomes less stable, so younger women tend to have healthier eggs than older women. A woman is born with all the eggs she will ever have, but usually only one is released each month during her reproductive life. So it's worth thinking about what those egg cells need to mature and be fertilized successfully.

Sperm and the environment

The sperm's head is full of genetic material. The mid-piece, or body, contains energy cells (powered by a sugary substance surrounding them) that drive the tail. Different parts of the sperm rely on different vitamins and minerals to work well (*see* pages 20–1). The seminal fluid that combines with sperm to form semen (about 20 percent of semen is sperm) is composed of a wide range of substances, including sugar, vitamins C, E and B$_{12}$, prostaglandins, zinc, potassium and sulfur, and essential fatty acids (namely DHA). Sperm are nourished by this liquid and it protects them from the acidic environment of a woman's vagina.

Sperm are produced constantly, and they are highly susceptible to environmental factors. Sperm counts have been steadily declining over the last 50 years, and scientific evidence points to exposure to chemicals and toxins as being a cause of this. Infertility has many causes, but insufficient emphasis is put on the importance of lifestyle factors to sperm quality. This can and should be addressed to optimize whatever fertility potential there is, for example by improving the diet. Sperm formation takes about 74 days, followed by another 20–30 days of maturation. So, once your partner has made changes to his lifestyle, he needs to allow about 100 days to see any improvement in sperm quality or quantity.

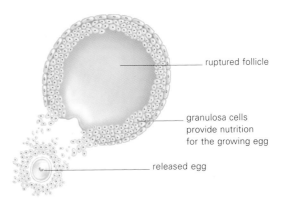

ruptured follicle

granulosa cells provide nutrition for the growing egg

released egg

Ovulation: it takes 150 days for an egg in a follicle in your ovary to develop into a mature egg ready to be released.

Fending off free radicals

Free radicals attack cells on a daily basis and damage both DNA and mitochondria. They are a natural by-product of our metabolism. But they are also produced by external agents when you smoke; when you eat processed foods; when you burn food; when you drink alcohol or take recreational drugs; and when you're exposed to environmental pollution.

In small quantities, and balanced by a nutritious diet full of antioxidants (*see* page 20), free radicals cause little harm, but if you are exposed to toxins on a daily basis and your diet is inadequate, they become a problem and can affect your fertility. Free radical damage is accumulative and increases with age.

BEING HORMONALLY HEALTHY

Hormonal balance is intrinsic to the functioning of our reproductive systems. People often don't make the link between what they eat and hormonal balance. Hormones are made from nutrients in food, so in order to have healthy sperm and eggs we need a digestive system that can break down and absorb vital nutrients. A diet that includes a lot of refined or junk foods causes hormonal havoc. Your aim, in choosing what to eat and drink, is to reduce the burden on your body, allowing all of its main systems—reproductive, circulatory, endocrine (hormone) and nervous—to function properly.

healthy eating

Eating healthily takes time, thought, and preparation, and to do it all the time is nearly impossible because of the hectic lifestyles we lead. It also depends on good digestion to maximize your body's absorption of vital nutrients, so start thinking about getting your digestive system healthy, ready for pregnancy.

IMPROVING DIGESTION

There are various ways you can help your digestive system become better able to absorb vital nutrients.
• Make time to eat and chew your food well.
• Don't drink water with meals—it dilutes the stomach's digestive juices—but drink lots of water, preferably filtered, throughout the day.
• Avoid eating raw foods late in the day.
• Don't eat carbohydrates late at night.
• Eat only until you are full.
• Aim for a 20 percent acid, 80 percent alkaline balance (*see* opposite page).

BLOOD-SUGAR LEVELS

Maintaining balanced blood-sugar levels is important. Low blood sugar causes symptoms such as headache, dizziness, fatigue, lack of energy, irritability, and cravings for sweet things. It also exacerbates premenstrual syndrome. If you eat refined carbohydrates (sugary foods such as cakes and cookies), they will be quickly digested, causing a rapid rise in the amount of glucose in your bloodstream. Insulin is then released to reduce the levels of glucose. This may lead to hypoglycemia (low blood sugar) and further fatigue and irritability, and cravings for sweet foods, as the whole cycle repeats.

In addition, refined carbohydrates contain no valuable nutrients and will cause you to gain weight. Since estrogen is stored in fat, weight gain

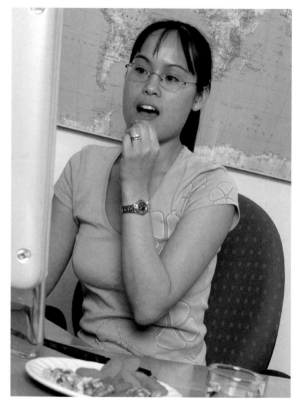

"balance your blood-sugar levels by eating little and often"

ACID-ALKALINE BALANCE

A woman's body needs to be alkaline for optimum fertility. Leading up to and around the time of ovulation, cervical secretions increase and these need to be alkaline to offer a good sperm environment. Your partner's sperm production also requires alkalinity.

The body's acid-alkaline balance needs to be 20-80 for optimum functioning, but our typical Western diet tends towards the reverse because we eat too much protein (acidic) and too little alkaline food. Protein is a necessary part of our diet, but it needs to be

balanced with lots of vegetables and fruits. A good acid-alkaline balance is easier to maintain than it is to achieve, so start to think about what category the foods you eat fall into and make long-term changes to your diet to get the balance right.

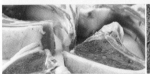 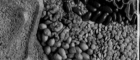 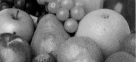 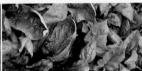

Strongly acidic foods	**Mildly acidic foods**	**Mildly alkaline foods**	**Strongly alkaline foods**
meat, fish, and carbonated drinks such as colas	grains, legumes, such as peas, beans, and lentils, and nuts	fruits, vegetables and dairy products	green leafy vegetables such as spinach and broccoli

will exacerbate any hormonal imbalance. This in turn affects the balance between estrogen and progesterone in the body. Normally, progesterone levels rise when estrogen levels drop after ovulation, and progesterone plays a part in conception, implantation, and the thickening of the womb lining. If estrogen levels remain high, secretion of progesterone will be affected. These hormone imbalances may affect your fertility.

Another consequence of yo-yoing blood-sugar levels is that, when levels drop, epinephrine is released. Elevated levels of stress hormones such as epinephrine also adversely affect hormone production.

To balance your blood-sugar levels, eat small amounts of wholesome food often. This will help your metabolism function properly and you will have more energy and no longer crave sweet foods. Make sure you:
• eat regularly—in particular, always eat breakfast.
• mix protein and carbohydrates in order to prolong the digestive process, balancing blood-sugar levels.
• eat complex carbohydrates such as wholewheat bread and pasta or oats.

SHOULD YOU DIET?

● I advise women who are overweight to try to slim down prior to pregnancy. But instead of dieting, I encourage them to eat healthily so that they will nourish their baby's growth and development without piling on the pounds. Your baby does not depend entirely on what you eat on any day; rather, it calls on your nutrient reserves, such as iron stored in bone marrow or folic acid in the liver.

● If you don't have adequate reserves because you have been restricting your food intake, and you continue to limit what you eat during pregnancy for fear of putting on too much weight, then you risk giving birth to a smaller baby whose potential for brain development has not been realized.

● Weight-loss programs that rely on high-protein, low-carbohydrate intakes are particularly bad for your health.

• eat lots of fresh fruit and lightly cooked fresh vegetables.
• snack on nuts and seeds.
• cut out refined carbohydrates—cakes, cookies, sweets, soft and carbonated drinks, white bread, white rice, white pasta, and white potatoes.

foundations of a staple diet

Take a careful look at what you eat on a daily basis. There are various components of a good diet that you should incorporate into your eating habits in preparation for pregnancy.

PROTEIN

Proteins are the building blocks of the body's cells and are vitally important for egg and sperm production. Proteins are made from 20 types of amino acids, most of which we can manufacture in our bodies, although there are eight that have to come from our diet and are known as essential amino acids. Animal proteins supply all the essential amino acids but plant sources do not.

Women need about 1¾oz (45g) of protein a day—about 15 percent of their daily calorie intake. Pregnant women need 2–2½oz (50–60g) and lactating women about 55g (2¼oz). Protein is essential for growth and repair of body cells. Make sure that you get an adequate amount when you are trying to conceive naturally or before IVF to facilitate the development of the egg.

Meat and fish are primary sources (that is, they contain a full range of amino acids), but we also get protein from dairy, produce, and vegetables such as legumes—peas, beans, and lentils. All fruit and vegetables contain varying amounts of protein —frozen peas and cooked spinach are particularly rich in protein. Red meat is more acidic than fish or chicken, so don't eat it more than once a week.

However, high-protein diets are not a good idea in the buildup to pregnancy. There is evidence that ammonia, which is a by-product of excessive protein metabolism, may interfere with embryo implantation. Too little protein, which may be the case with vegetarians (*see* page 46), can also be detrimental. You may become deficient in vitamins B_2 and B_6, which are needed to neutralize acidity. A diet too low in protein can also hinder hormone release.

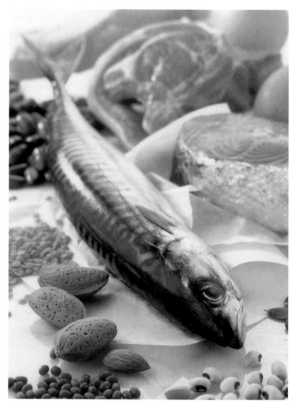

Eating a variety of foods that are rich sources of protein ensures a good balance of all 20 amino acids in your diet.

CARBOHYDRATE

Carbohydrates are valuable energy foods, but what is important is the type of carbohydrates you eat and the balance within your diet. Complex carbohydrates, which release energy gradually, are better foods than simple carbohydrates, which cause fluctuations in blood-sugar levels that affect the functioning of body systems (*see* pages 16–17).

Carbohydrate metabolism results in alcohol production. Simple carbohydrates produce alcohols that can be toxic to the body, and highly refined foods are acid producers. Include in your diet complex carbohydrates such as legumes, grains, and wholewheat breads and pasta.

DO I NEED VITAMIN AND MINERAL SUPPLEMENTS?

Food is the best source of nutrients for the body and we should get all the vitamins and minerals we need from eating a healthy diet. However, because of the lifestyles we lead, most of us would benefit from a good multivitamin and mineral supplement. I believe this becomes all the more important when you are trying to conceive and during pregnancy—so ask your pharmacist to recommend a reputable brand of supplement containing the appropriate amounts of necessary nutrients.

● Research has shown that the chances of a couple conceiving and carrying a baby to term may be increased by taking a supplement. Supplements have also been shown to reduce the risk of low birth weight and certain fetal abnormalities.

● If your prenatal supplement does not contain 400 mcg of folic acid, your doctor can prescribe it. Folic acid taken during conception and pregnanacy helps reduce the risk of neural tube defects in the fetus (see page 59).

● Remember that supplements are not a solution to an inadequate diet; you may need to make other lifestyle changes to ensure optimum health in pregnancy.

The secret to good carbohydrate intake is to avoid eating carbs late in the day, when they will stay longer in the system, allowing more time for the production of alcohols, which need to be detoxified and eliminated from the body. Ideally, you should eat complex carbohydrates with protein because this prolongs the digestive process so that energy is released over a longer period of time.

FAT

There is now much evidence to demonstrate the importance of essential fatty acids (EFAs) for health, reproduction, and fetal development. EFAs are important for hormonal balance, the immune system, and ovary, egg, and sperm health, yet our bodies are unable to make them and it is difficult for us to get an adequate amount from our diet. Eight out of ten women are deficient in EFAs and it takes up to three months to build up reserves in the body systems. Unless you are eating 1oz (30g) of nuts and seeds a day and 10oz (300g) of oily fish a week you are unlikely to be getting enough, and with the ongoing debate about how many fish to eat in light of fears over contamination with mercury, I feel that supplements are a good alternative. Start taking a fish oil supplement containing omega-3 and omega-6 essential fatty acids when you start planning your pregnancy and continue throughout pregnancy and beyond.

WATER

Drinking water not only keeps you hydrated, it maintains good blood circulation, which is important for the transportation of nutrients and hormones, and to maintain blood pressure. Although we get liquid from food and drinks such as tea and coffee, water should be part of our daily liquid intake.

When water is in short supply, the body ensures that the organs vital for life receive what they need at the expense of other body systems such as the reproductive system. But adequate hydration is important here, too, for good cervical mucus, plump follicles, and a strong blood supply to the uterine lining so that it can nurture a fertilized egg. The same goes for sperm health and motility: adequate hydration is necessary for the production of prostatic fluid (one of the constituents of semen) and to help prevent clumping of sperm.

Although tap water is safe to drink, it often contains added fluoride, high levels of which can affect the functioning of your thyroid and consequently have an impact on fertility. Chlorine can also be harmful. If you fill a pitcher with tap water and leave it for awhile, most of the chlorine will evaporate. If you filter your water, using a carbonated filter, you will improve its quality and taste. Bottled water varies: some mineral waters are high in sodium, while others are beneficial because they include magnesium and calcium.

nutrients for conception

When you are trying to conceive a baby, various nutrients are particularly important for egg and sperm quality, implantation, and development of the embryo. Some of these vital nutrients are listed here; their food sources can be found on pages 134–7.

ANTIOXIDANTS

Certain nutrients—vitamins A, C, and E, selenium, zinc, manganese, and copper, for example—act as antioxidants and protect body cells against free radical damage (*see* page 15). Your body produces some antioxidants naturally, but others, such as vitamins, must come from your diet. The recommendation in the food pyramid, of five portions of fruit and vegetables a day, is one way of ensuring an adequate intake of antioxidants.

Different nutrients have different roles: vitamin C protects against free radical damage in the blood;

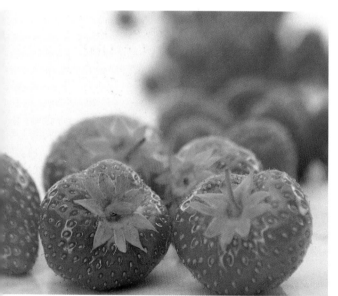

Antioxidants found in fruit are essential for the protection of body cells against damage by toxins such as free radicals.

vitamin E and other fat-soluble antioxidants protect fatty structures such as cell membranes; and co-enzyme Q_{10} helps support the mitochondria, the powerhouses of all cells. Women considering pregnancy are now advised not to take supplements containing more than 5,000 IU of vitamin A because an excess can cause birth defects.

B VITAMINS

All B vitamins are essential for ovulation and implantation. B vitamins are also important for hormonal control and fetal development. Because they are water soluble they are quickly lost from the body, and lifestyle factors such as stress and drinking alcohol can cause your reserves to become depleted.

FOLIC ACID

Folic acid is a B vitamin that helps prevent birth defects of the spinal cord and brain called neural tube defects (NTDs; *see* page 59), which result in spina bifida and anencephaly. NTDs happen in the first month of pregnancy, so you need to make sure you have enough folic acid in your system before you conceive. Start taking folic acid when trying to conceive and continue throughout pregnancy because levels drop in the second and third trimesters due to changes in your blood folate level.

Folate is the natural form of folic acid found in foods such as legumes and leafy green vegetables. However, the body absorbs folic acid from supplements and fortified foods more readily than it does from food.

Homocysteine

People with a low dietary intake of folate, vitamins B$_{12}$ and B$_6$, zinc, or magnesium sometimes have high levels of homocysteine, an amino acid that is produced by the body. If levels of homocysteine are elevated in pregnancy, there is an increased risk of miscarriage and preeclampsia.

CALCIUM

Most cells in the body use calcium. Not only does it keep bones and teeth strong and healthy, it helps maintain the circulatory, muscular, and nervous systems. If you do not get enough calcium from your diet, your body will take it from stores in your bones, which, over time, might become weakened. Although the recommended amount of calcium is 1,000mg a day, the average daily intake of women of childbearing age is only about 700mg. If you don't get enough calcium in your diet, check that there is an adequate amount in your supplement.

DHA

An essential component of the brain, eyes and nerve cells is docosahexaenoic acid (DHA), an omega-3 essential fatty acid (*see* page 19), which the body uses for specific functions. This fatty acid makes up 60 percent of an adult's brain weight and 20 percent of a baby's.

In women, the first pregnancy-related need for fatty acids occurs during the three months before conception, when cells in the ovaries are dividing. Healthy, viable eggs need DHA to grow and develop. DHA is also an important nutrient during pregnancy, for lowering the mother's blood pressure and prolonging gestation as well as ensuring the development of the growing fetus (*see* page 59).

According to Professor Michael Crawford of the Institute of Brain Chemistry at the University of North London, "DHA is the backbone of the brain's signaling structures. It plays an especially important part in the growth and development of the fetal brain and during a baby's first six months of life."

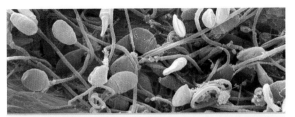

NUTRIENTS FOR HEALTHY SPERM

There are certain nutrients that are especially important for the health of sperm. See pages 134–7 for food sources.

Vitamin C Protects sperm from oxidative damage and improves sperm quality in men who smoke. Men who have a condition known as agglutination, in which sperm clump together, may benefit from vitamin C supplements.

Zinc An insufficiency of zinc, often called the "fertility mineral", is believed to lead to a reduced sperm count and erectile dysfunction. Needed to make the outer layer and tail of sperm, it is lost with each ejaculation, so an active sex life and a low-zinc diet place a man at risk of reduced fertility.

Vitamin B$_{12}$ This is necessary to maintain fertility. Studies have shown an improvement in sperm count after injections of vitamin B$_{12}$, and in sperm motility when vitamin B$_{12}$ is taken orally.

Selenium This is an essential trace mineral that has antioxidant properties and may improve sperm motility.

Arginine This amino acid is needed for sperm production. Supplements may increase sperm count and quality as well as enhancing the immune system, stimulating growth hormones, and maintaining circulation (and hence sexual function).

DHA DHA is highly concentrated in the testes and may regulate enzymes in the process of making sperm. Semen contains high levels of DHA, which appears to be needed to energize sperm and increase their motility.

Coenzyme Q$_{10}$ This nutrient is used by the cells to produce energy and may have a role in sperm production. There is evidence that supplements improve both sperm count and motility.

looking at your lifestyle

Before actively trying to conceive a baby, look at what I call your lifestyle factors and those of your partner to see if anything might compromise conception and pregnancy. Most of us have a lot of demands placed upon us—think about what you can change in your lives to improve your overall well-being.

WHAT SHOULD YOU CHANGE?

When you start planning to become pregnant ask yourself the following questions to establish whether or not your lifestyle needs to change.

Do you drink a lot of alcohol?

A by-product of alcohol metabolism is acetaldehyde, which is toxic to sperm, so bear in mind the 100-day cycle of sperm production (*see* page 15) and start to cut back right away.

Control your drinking. People who drink heavily also tend to have a poor diet. Not only does alcohol deplete their B vitamins, for example, but they tend not to eat properly. And, since alcoholic drinks are high in calories, they are fattening, too. Also, beware succumbing to the temptations of binge drinking as a misguided remedy for stress.

I usually say that the odd glass of wine while you are trying to conceive does no harm, but I do advise you to stop drinking alcohol between ovulation and your next period, when you may not be aware you have conceived. Once you are pregnant, I advise no alcohol at all (*see* page 43).

Do you smoke?

If either you or your partner smoke, now is the time to stop. Smoking doubles the amount of free radical damage in your body, while robbing it of nutrients that are essential to the development of eggs and sperm. Smoking also increases intakes

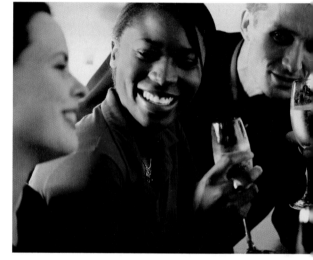

An occasional drink while trying to conceive does no harm, and a night out with friends can be a good stress reliever.

of lead and cadmium, both of which are highly toxic, and reduces oxygen intake, making cell replication less efficient.

Men who smoke are likely to have decreased sperm density; less motile sperm; more abnormal sperm; lower testosterone levels; and children with an increased risk of developing cancer. The concentration of sperm among male smokers is 17 percent lower than among nonsmokers.

Smoking nearly doubles a woman's risk of having a low-birthweight baby. Nicotine constricts blood vessels in the uterus, which decreases the

HOW WELL DO YOU SLEEP?

● I always stress the importance of sleep in balancing body systems and building up energy reserves. While our bodies can manage physically with little sleep, our brains cannot. Switching off conscious brain activity when we sleep is essential for brain health and functioning.

● Sleep really energizes us, so getting a good work and rest balance is important. If you find you are regularly eating late, going to bed late, and getting up early, you are not building up your sleep reserves.

● Sleep is a restorative mechanism. It gives your body a break and enables it to rebalance. When planning a pregnancy, you need to take a careful look at your lifestyle and start to get into positive sleeping habits. For example, try to go to bed at the same time every evening (preferably before 11pm) and get up at the same time every morning—this allows your body to get into a regular rhythm.

● We all have an internal body clock, or circadian rhythm, that functions roughly on a 24-hour cycle and governs bodily functions—it dictates whether we feel sleepy or wakeful, energized or tired, and when we need food, as well as controlling fluctuations in body temperature and hormone secretions. We are essentially diurnal creatures, which means we function during daylight hours and sleep when it's dark.

● Knowing when these rhythms occur allows us to work with them rather than against them. Going to bed without feeling exhausted actually helps us sleep better: it allows time to relax, switch off, and achieve better quality sleep.

blood supply to your fetus, reducing the oxygen available. It is also linked to a number of pregnancy complications, such as premature rupturing of membranes and problems with the placenta.

Do you use drugs?

When it comes to sperm production, persistent use of cannabis is bad news. Its active ingredient, tetrahydrocannabinol, increases the number of sperm with abnormal head shapes, thereby making it harder for them to fertilize an egg. The chemical is also toxic to the developing egg.

If you use cocaine it can seriously affect your chance of conceiving a baby. It binds to sperm, making them less motile, and it causes problems at fertilization, when the sperm try to penetrate an egg. Women who use cocaine risk growth retardation of their babies in utero and increase the risk of giving birth prematurely.

Are you the correct weight?

If you're very overweight, you're likely to be less fertile; you'll have an increased risk of miscarrying; and there are more likely to be complications during your pregnancy. Losing just 10 percent of your body weight can restore hormone balance. Being seriously underweight may affect ovulation and estrogen production. If you do conceive, you might not produce enough hormones for the pregnancy to continue. Too few fat cells means too little estrogen, which can affect cervical secretions, too. Menstrual periods cease altogether if you fall below a certain weight.

In men, sperm quality is affected and sperm production will cease if you are 25 percent below normal body weight for height (*see* below).

CALCULATING YOUR BMI

To see if you're the right weight for your height, calculate your BMI (body mass index). Divide your weight in pounds by your height in inches squared, and multiply by 703. For example, a woman who is 5ft 7in (1.7m) tall and 138lb (65kg) would calculate her BMI as follows:

$$143lb \div (67in \times 67in) \times 703 = 22.4\ BMI$$

Your BMI should be between 19 and 25. Less than 19 means you are underweight; more than 25 means you are overweight.

are you fit for pregnancy?

Many women are concerned about exercise. How much and what type should they do? When should they do it? Should they stop when they are ovulating? I think the answers to such questions often depend on factors such as the type of exercise you do, your bodyweight, and the level of exertion to which you are accustomed. But I think the most important thing is to enjoy whatever exercise you choose to do.

BENEFITS OF EXERCISE

Regular exercise makes you feel more positive, and prevents depression as natural endorphins are released. It also improves your circulation and gives you energy, making you feel less sluggish.

However, most of us lead sedentary lives and don't do enough regular exercise. As a result, everything from our breathing (hence oxygen levels) to our lymphatic circulation (hence detoxification) is negatively affected.

Fortunately, this can be rectified quite easily. If you exercise for 20–30 minutes a day, you will start to notice an improvement in how you feel within a month. The important thing is to find a form of exercise you enjoy, that suits you, and that can be built into your daily routine.

On the other side of the coin, I see couples who are fanatics about exercise, to the point where they do it rigorously every day. There is evidence that too much exercise impacts on fertility. Sperm production may decrease, and female hormones may be suppressed. As with all things, balance is key.

RELAXATION

Many of the couples I see find it very hard to relax. In many cases, they see relaxation as being part of their exercise routine, rather than an opportunity to take time out to sit and read a book, or go and see friends. Their lives operate around a busy schedule and they feel uncomfortable when

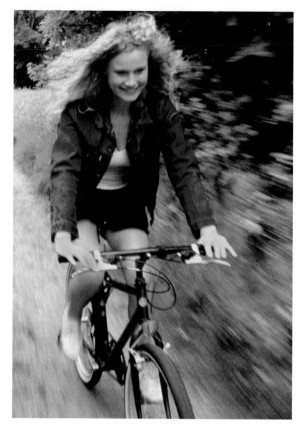

Regular exercise helps relieve stress and tension. Choose an activity you enjoy so that you will want to do it regularly.

there is no pressure. However, for the sake of good health, it is necessary to figure out a way of making sure you do enjoy some relaxation time.

Constant tension exacerbates a wide range of physical problems, from raised blood pressure to irritable bowel syndrome. When we feel tense, our bodies produce hormones such as epinephrine and cortisol (*see* pages 26–7), which prepare us for action. The result is tense muscles that are difficult to relax, so much so that tension in our bodies becomes impossible to shift without external help such as a massage. Try to avoid this by incorporating regular exercise and relaxation into your daily life.

How relaxed you are will have a direct effect on the state of your muscles. Practicing simple relaxation techniques will help you recognize when your muscles are tense and when they are relaxed. Tense muscles restrict blood flow and hence limit oxygen supply. Inadequate oxygen results in a buildup of lactic acid in the muscles and can make them susceptible to damage. Persistently high levels of lactic acid can result in an acidic state within the body that isn't healthy (*see* page 17).

If you've been stressed for awhile, learning to relax may take some time. You may need to do physical activity beforehand to free the muscles of some of the tension. Alternatively, take a long bath by candlelight, listen to music, immerse yourself in a good book, or go for a solitary walk. What is important is to find something that works for you, and then integrate it into your life. If stress has become a problem, you may need help. Many of my clients find hypnotherapy helps them achieve a relaxed state and they can be shown how to do it themselves (*see* page 103).

Breathing

We breathe automatically, from the moment we are born until we die. But breathing is also something we can influence at will, and this gives us a powerful tool. When I talk to clients about having a session on learning how to breathe, they look surprised. We no longer breathe as we did as babies, and we carry a lot of tension with us as a result. However, we can learn to breathe in a way that influences our physical, psychological, and spiritual well-being.

Most of us breathe shallowly, using the top part of our chest, as if we are prepared for "flight or fight" (*see* page 26). This creates unrelieved tension in the chest, which spreads into our shoulders, neck, forehead, and face, and also restricts abdominal organs. According to many stress experts, learning to breathe properly (*see* box below) is the most important tool available for relaxation and stress management. Diaphragmatic breathing also relieves constriction of the large intestine, which helps release a tense gut and its associated problems.

BREATHING CORRECTLY

1 Lie on your back with your knees bent and your back flat on the floor.
2 Relax your shoulders, and tuck your chin in so your neck is long. A small cushion under your head is fine.
3 Gently rest one hand on your upper chest and one on your abdomen.
4 Close your eyes and breathe gently and regularly, in through the nose, out through the mouth.
5 Notice your chest rising. Take each breath a little deeper into the abdomen so you feel your ribs expanding and your abdomen extending slightly.
6 Place your hands by your sides, and continue breathing in this way.

7 As your breathing becomes calmer and more efficient, you should find you are breathing, naturally, between 12 and 16 times a minute, less as you relax.

Practice for 10 minutes, two or three times a day, until this way of breathing becomes automatic whether you are

lying, sitting, or standing. Sometimes it helps to intone the word "in" on an inhalation, and "out" on an exhalation. This helps focus your mind and prevent unwelcome thoughts from crowding in. If you are still finding it hard to switch off, try visualization (*see* page 67).

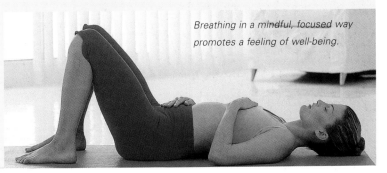

Breathing in a mindful, focused way promotes a feeling of well-being.

how stressed are you?

There's no doubt that we all feel stressed from time to time. A degree of stress is an inevitable part of life, but when it becomes a constant feature of our daily routine, it causes problems. I see countless women who are worrying that they are too stressed to conceive a baby.

WHAT IS STRESS?

There is much new research available on how stress can affect the fetus and also on how stress in the womb affects your child's ability to deal with stress in later

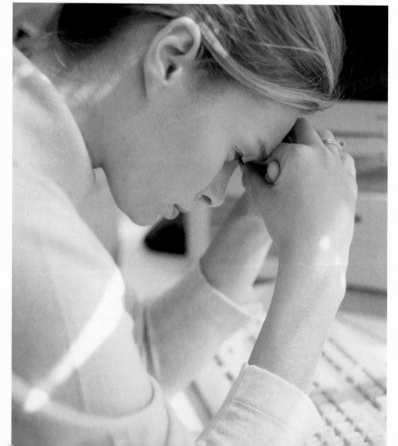

life. I believe it is vitally important to learn how to recognize and manage your stress levels before you conceive.

Today, we have a great need to be in control of our lives,

and when we lose control, we are unable to handle the stress. People who are constantly thinking are using up energy.

It is hard sometimes to know that you are stressed. You are probably not even aware until you notice that your muscles are tense and your breathing is shallow. Chronic stress leads to the hormones epinephrine and cortisol being released ready for fight or flight. However, if your body keeps cortisol levels permanently raised, you will become exhausted, finding it hard to relax and sleep and unable to build up your reserves. This eventually leads to anxiety and depression.

Having stress hormones permanently in the body is toxic because they take their toll on the endocrine and immune systems, and also deplete your nutritional reserves. Too little cortisol, on the other hand, results in muscular weakness and an inability to mobilize energy in times of high demand.

THE BRAIN UNDER STRESS

Once you are pregnant, one of the most dramatic effects of the stress hormone cortisol is on fetal brain development and the way the brain circuits are put together, determining how the child reacts to stress in later life.

Researchers have found that if there are higher cortisol levels in the fetus, the brain becomes programmed to tolerate them. This can then result in higher, more harmful levels being tolerated in stressful situations later in life.

You can see then how important it is to control your stress response before and during pregnancy—bear in mind that a pregnancy does not last forever, but the effects of a negative womb environment can last a lifetime.

CAUSES OF STRESS

A manageeable amount of stress can be a good thing—it is when you start to feel overwhelmed that it becomes a problem. A little stress is also good for your fetus, but it is when the stress levels are high and constant over many days and weeks that it may have permanent effects on the developing brain.

Chronic stress factors include financial concerns, the death of a close relative or friend, relationships with aging parents, stepchildren, or partners from previous relationships. Working long hours is stressful and often

goes hand in hand with poor eating habits, lack of sleep, and little sex.

The couples I see, especially if they are having problems conceiving, deal with a lot of stress as they experience a roller-coaster of emotions—worry, fear, anger, grief, joy. The women in particular are often worried. Will my pregnancy test be positive? Will I have another miscarriage? What if I never get pregnant?

Many women lose faith in their body's ability to do the right thing, but, in fact, the body is always trying to restore equilibrium in its internal systems, despite variations in external conditions.

RESTORING BALANCE

So how do you know if your systems are out of balance? You need to look carefully at your lifestyle and identify potential trouble spots. For example, is your work load too big? If the

answer is yes, look at ways of cutting it down. Start to analyze the problems and see how they can be addressed. Learn how to reduce your stress levels, conserve your energy, and take time out whenever you get the chance. Getting rid of physical tension through exercise will help you reduce emotional tension.

The Chinese believe that the way to restore balance in the body and build up reserves of energy is to sleep, breathe deeply (see page 25), and meditate.

If you feel stressed by life in general, imagine how much more stressed you might feel if pregnancy doesn't occur just when you have planned. Think also about the effects high stress levels might have on your baby once you are pregnant. And consider how stressful life might be once you are juggling the demands of a young family. Start your stress management now!

ARE YOU CHRONICALLY STRESSED?

If you answer yes to any of the following questions, it might indicate a state of chronic stress, which you need to address.

- Do you often find it difficult to fall asleep?
- Are you restless during the night?
- Do you wake during the early hours, then find you can't get back to sleep?
- Do you find it difficult to relax when you have time off?
- Are you fidgety and restless when you try to relax?
- Do you suffer from indigestion?
- Do you often feel mildly nauseous?
- Do you crave coffee and other stimulants?
- Do you forget what you've just gone to find?
- Do you often feel grumpy, tired, and irritable?
- Are you prone to tearfulness?

environmental impact

Until recently, scientists paid little attention to the effects of environmental agents on human reproduction, but a lot of research has been done on animals, revealing that chemicals do have an impact in particular on male reproduction, affecting the testes or damaging the sperm themselves.

POTENTIAL HAZARDS

Abnormalities in an embryo are a major cause of early miscarriage: they prevent normal development and the embryo dies. While this was previously thought to be a fault with the woman's egg, or a random mutation, it is becoming evident that abnormalities in sperm may be a contributing factor. Although abnormalities may be inherited, they can also be caused by environmental pollutants and lifestyle factors such as smoking. Sperm are particularly vulnerable to this because they are in constant production.

In early pregnancy, your environment can have a profound impact on a developing embryo. From day 15 to day 60 – that is, the second to the eighth week, known as the embryonic period – is a critical time for the development of your baby's organs and it may be the case that you do not even know you are pregnant for some of this time.

Don't start panicking, but be aware when you have a baby on board that certain substances pass through the placenta (*see* page 57). There are more than four million chemical mixtures in homes and businesses that may affect a fetus, as well as environmental pollutants in air and water.

Around the house

Many products are potentially hazardous. Be especially wary of household cleansers, paints, varnishes, air fresheners, carpet cleaners, dry-cleaning fluids, printing inks, equipment, or furnishings containing flame retardants and stain removers. You should also be conscious of beauty products such as hair dyes, nail polish, and varnish, fragrances, and deodorants. Many of these contain organic solvents (chemicals that dissolve other substances), which give off fumes. Phythalates and parabens are chemicals that are used in some makeup products and toiletries, yet both are

EVERYDAY TECHNOLOGY

Much debate continues about the effects of computers, mobile phones and microwaves on health. Try to limit their use when planning or during a pregnancy.

● There has been a lot of concern about visual display units (VDUs) causing miscarriage or birth defects. But extensive research has so far shown this not to be the case. However, it's probably a good idea not to sit for hours with a laptop on your knee—and this applies to men as well as women.

● The jury is still out on cell phones and much more research is needed on long-term safety. So, carry your phone in a bag rather than putting it in your pocket, and keep it away from your abdomen.

● In the home, limit your use of the microwave and don't stand in front of it while it's operating. You might also want to avoid using an electric blanket while you're trying to conceive; use a down comforter instead. Take a hot water bottle to bed or keep each other warm instead.

suspected of disrupting the hormonal balance, so get into the habit of checking labels carefully for chemical content.

When gardening, do not use powerful weedkillers or any other chemicals and wear gloves to reduce the risk of catching toxoplasmosis (*see* page 47). If you have hobbies such as painting and enameling, use products with caution. To put it simply, if you or your partner are doing anything around the house that involves powerful chemicals, limit your exposure, ventilate the room well, and wear protective clothes.

Metals to avoid

Lead is found in decreasing amounts in industry and manufacturing, but may still be found in the piping of old houses and lead crystal glassware. Recent research shows that lead in sperm prevents it from binding to the egg. Lead has also been linked to stillbirths because deposits of lead have been found in the placenta. Vitamin C may assist in the removal of lead from the body, as well as pectin, found in apples, pears, and bananas.

You can be exposed to mercury by eating contaminated fish. While trace amounts are present in most fish, it is most concentrated in large species. I now recommend supplements to replace the important nutrients, such as essential fatty acids, that we need from fish. Avoid having mercury dental fillings put in or removed while you are trying to conceive.

Other metals to be wary of are cadmium (cigarettes, fertilizers, processed foods), aluminum (saucepans, foil, food additives), and copper (jewelry, IUDs, water pipes—use a water filter).

Pesticides

Avoid pesticides as much as possible. Research has shown that exposure to these may contribute to miscarriage, premature birth, and birth defects. (A study published in *The Lancet* in 1994 found that organic farmers had much higher sperm counts than farmers using chemicals.) Some pesticides,

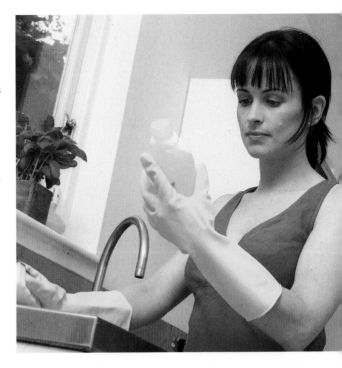

"get into the habit of checking product labels carefully"

known as endocrine disruptors, have estrogen-like qualities that may affect the reproductive system of a fetus. Wash all fruit and vegetables, wear rubber gloves when gardening, and avoid insect repellents containing DEET.

Other chemicals

Polychlorinated biphenyls (PCBs) are mixtures of chemicals that are no longer used in manufacturing of electrical equipment but can still be released into the environment from hazardous waste sites or leaks. They do not break down readily. PCBs have been linked to reproductive problems and impaired development in the womb as well as to cancer.

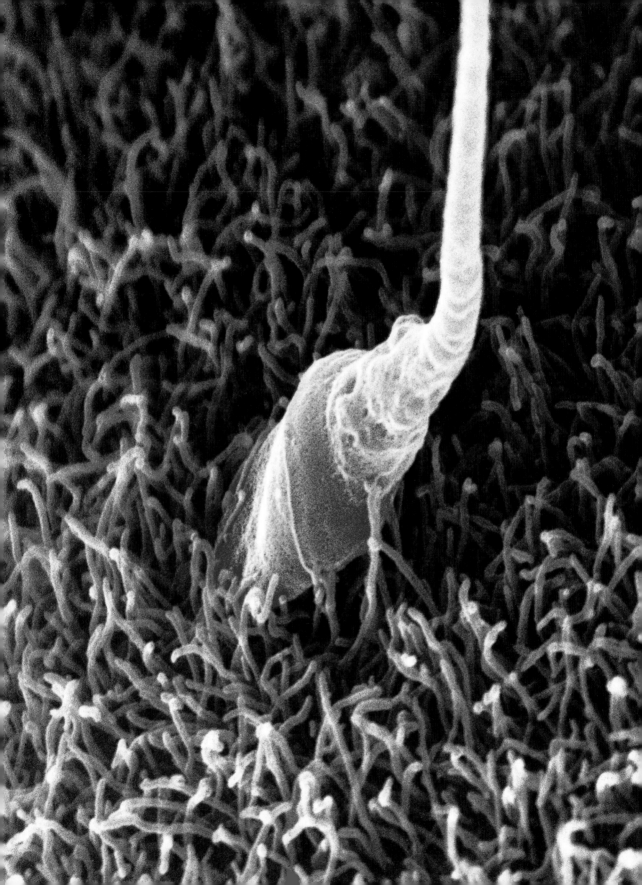

CONCEIVING A BABY

ovulation and fertilization

It takes 150 days to "grow" an egg. Follicles (small sacs containing eggs) begin to form, then one starts to develop faster, becoming dominant. A complex interplay of hormones allows the egg to mature and be released. The timing of ovulation varies from woman to woman, but it's usually two weeks after a period.

EGG CATCHING

Once released, the egg is "caught" by the fallopian tube. Tiny hairlike cells guide the egg into the tube where it remains, anticipating fertilization, for about 48 hours. Meanwhile, the mature follicle that released the egg still has a role to play, as a tissue mass called the corpus luteum. Having secreted estrogen, it now releases progesterone, which prepares the outer cell layer of the uterine lining to receive a fertilized egg.

THE INCREDIBLE JOURNEY

Upon ejaculation, 250 million sperm race to the egg. The fastest, strongest, and those that take the shortest route will get there first—some in as little as 30 minutes. The secretions a woman produces each month are alkaline and have channels for sperm to swim up. In the absence of these the environment is too acidic and sperm will die. Usually, sperm survive for three to five days.

SPERM MEETS EGG

Sperm must first get through the nutrients surrounding an egg to reach the outer "shell." They have to be strong—only a few hundred

One in 250 million: a sperm reaches and fertilizes the waiting egg ahead of its many competitors.

will make it. It can take hours for them to get through the shell, which is hard and difficult to penetrate. A sperm has a drill-like action. As it passes through the shell, it sheds its protective head covering. The successful sperm swim into the fluid space surrounding the egg. The nucleus containing the woman's genetic information is found inside the egg. Several sperm will get into the narrow area between the shell and the membrane, but only one can penetrate it.

The man's genes are in the sperm head; once inside the egg, the head swells and becomes a nucleus, so now there are two nuclei in the egg. They draw together, fuse, and a unique individual is created.

BOY OR GIRL?

The sex of a baby is determined at the point of fertilization by the sperm. There are two sex chromosomes—X and Y. Females have a pair of Xs and males have an X and a Y. In preparation for fertilization, an egg loses one of its pair, and as sperm mature they carry only an X or a Y. So, when the genetic material of egg and sperm fuses, either an XX or an XY offspring is produced. Some people believe that couples can determine the sex of their baby by timing sex, but I don't think there is much evidence to support this.

the first seven days

The time it takes between the moment of fertilization and the attachment of a fertilized egg to the lining of the uterus is usually about seven days.

DAY 1

The genetic material of the father and mother combine as the two nuclei fuse. Once fertilization is complete a single cell is formed from which the millions of body cells of the baby will develop. A newly fertilized egg is called a zygote. Within 12 hours the single cell divides, creating an exact copy of itself. The fertilized egg is still surrounded by nutrient cells, and nutrients pass through the cell membrane, providing nourishment.

DAYS 2–5

As the developing ball of embryonic cells is propelled slowly toward the uterus, cell division continues. The number of cells doubles roughly every 12 hours. The fertilized egg travels through the fallopian tube for another three days. Forty-eight hours after fertilization there are four cells; then eight, and so on, and they quickly become hard to distinguish. These cells are called stem cells and they will eventually evolve into the 200 different types of cells making up every part of the human body. The fertilized egg is now called a morula.

DAYS 5–6

After another day a hollow, where cell division is taking place and the embryo is forming, becomes visible, and the morula becomes a blastocyst. It is at this point that the first clear division of purpose among cells can be detected. The outer wall of the blastocyst is called the trophoblast and this will develop into the placenta and the membranes that cover the fetus. The inner mass of cells will develop into the embryo.

The blastocyst has found its way to the narrow part at the end of the fallopian tube and entered the womb. It floats around in search of a place to embed. Should the blastocyst get stuck in this narrow part it can result in an ectopic pregnancy, where the embryo embeds in the fallopian tube.

DAYS 6–7

Just before the blastocyst lands, the embryo expands and then sheds its shell. This is known as hatching. Whereas before, the outside of the blastocyst was smooth, the new surface of the embryo is ribbed and sticky. From now on it grows quickly as it searches for a suitable landing site in the uterine lining. Raised areas of the mucous membrane send out chemical signals that act like a kind of beacon to the embryo.

Most embryos embed on the upper back wall of the uterus. As soon as embryo and lining make contact, the cells that will form the placenta penetrate the membrane and there begins an exchange of chemical signals, nutrients, and oxygen. Soon hormonal signals from the rapidly developing placenta alert the woman's body systems to the fact that a fetus has started to grow in her uterus.

IVF AND CELL DIVISION

If you are undergoing IVF (*see* pages 38–9), you will be very aware of the different stages of cell division. Once the eggs are extracted, you have to wait to hear about the progress of fertilization and cell division. When the embryos are put back depends on your clinic: some are put back at two days and some are left for five days. In the case of older women, the outside of the egg capsule is often harder, so the embryo has more difficulty hatching successfully. Your consultant may suggest a technique known as assisted hatching, which helps the embryo break out of the shell.

Once fertilized, the egg begins a remarkable journey during which it divides and changes many times, before it finally reaches its eventual destination, the uterus, where it implants.

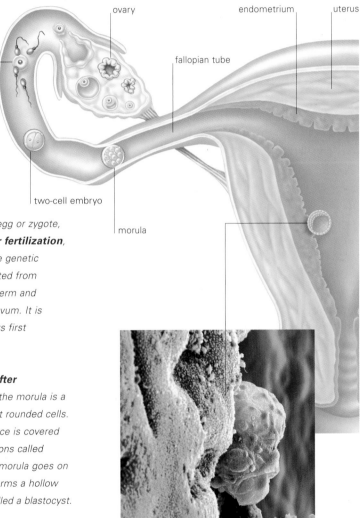

ovary

endometrium

uterus

fallopian tube

two-cell embryo

morula

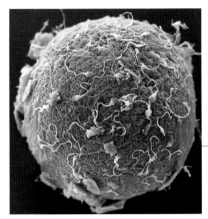

Fertilization: sperm (blue) can be seen attempting to penetrate an egg (red). Each sperm has a rounded head and a long tail.

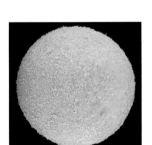

This fertilized egg or zygote, **one day after fertilization**, contains all the genetic material inherited from the father's sperm and the mother's ovum. It is preparing for its first cell division.

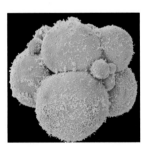

Three days after fertilization, the morula is a cluster of eight rounded cells. Each cell surface is covered in tiny projections called microvilli. The morula goes on dividing and forms a hollow ball of cells called a blastocyst.

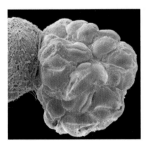

Six to seven days after fertilization, the blastocyst hatches before implanting. Most of its cells will form the placenta and membranes around the embryo, and only a small group form the embryo itself.

Once it reaches the uterus, **usually about seven days after fertilization**, the embryo prepares to implant in the womb lining. Most embryos implant on the upper back wall of the uterus, where the placenta will not block the cervix when the time for birth arrives.

when pregnancy fails

Many women get pregnant each month without even knowing it has happened. Then they may experience heavier bleeding than their usual period because the embryo has failed to implant and the pregnancy fails. A lot of current research is focused on why implantation sometimes does not occur.

FAILURE TO IMPLANT

The moment of implantation is critical, and many embryos fail to implant. Several factors come into play in determining whether or not implantation occurs. First, the uterine lining (endometrium) has to be healthy and thick in order to give the embryo a good root system—the way a plant relies on nourishment from the soil. Another major factor is the role of the immune system. A fertilized egg is like a foreign protein in the body, and there follows a delicate interplay between the uterine lining and cells in the embryo (trophoblasts) that will later become the placenta. They "communicate" to see whether the uterine lining will allow the embryo to embed.

Many women have problems with implantation these days, and it is my belief that, with so many chemicals in our food and in our environment, our immune systems are struggling to cope on all fronts. I believe that by detoxifying and de-stressing our bodies and building up reserves through sleep, exercise, and good nutrition, we can relieve the pressure and encourage the body's natural ability to rebalance itself. You can assist the process further with acupuncture, visualization (*see* page 67), or meditation (*see* page 81).

NATURAL TIPS FOR THICKENING YOUR UTERINE LINING

The uterine lining should be 9–10mm thick prior to implantation. A poor uterine lining may be the result of a previous uterine infection, hormonal imbalance such as low progesterone, or fibroids. Try the following:

● Take supplements of the antioxidant vitamins C and E and selenium to guard against free-radical damage.

● Eat foods containing bioflavonoids, such as citrus fruits, broccoli, grapes, and tomatoes. These have antioxidant properties and will improve blood flow.

● Take a vitamin B₁ supplement and make sure your diet is rich in this vitamin to improve blood supply and build up your uterine lining.

● Eat foods rich in essential fatty acids, iron, and protein: include nuts, spinach, seeds, garlic, and oatmeal in your diet (*see* pages 134–7).

● Arginine, an amino acid, has also been shown to improve the uterine lining. Take it as a supplement.

● Acupuncture may improve blood flow to the endometrium.

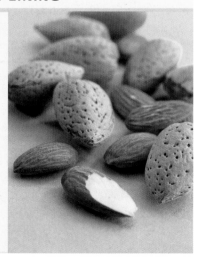

WHAT IS A MISCARRIAGE?

A miscarriage is defined as the loss of a pregnancy during the first 24 weeks of gestation. Most miscarriages occur during the first 12 weeks. About half of all fertilized eggs are unable to continue to a viable pregnancy.

Miscarriage happens for many different reasons, but I believe that by balancing your immune system, improving your nutrition and lifestyle preconceptually, and boosting your antioxidant status (*see* page 20), you can significantly reduce the risk.

CAUSES OF MISCARRIAGE

There are many reasons why women miscarry.
• **Genetics** The most common cause of a single (not recurrent) miscarriage is an abnormality in the chromosomes of the egg or the sperm.
• **Hormones** This may be because low progesterone levels prevent implantation and cause hormonal imbalance; or the levels of the hormone that stimulates the follicles to release eggs (follicle-stimulating hormone, FSH) are too high.
• **Infection** Some infections in pregnancy, such as sexually transmitted diseases and viral infections, make you more susceptible to miscarriage.
• **Abnormal anatomy** This could be a distortion of the uterus, scar tissue caused by previous surgery or infection, or, beyond 14 weeks, cervical incompetence, which means that the cervix does not remain closed during pregnancy.
• **Blood disorders** Some women are more prone to blood disorders, which make them more liable to miscarry.
• **Immunological disorders** (*see* right) Failure of IVF, as well as recurrent miscarriage, are now reasons to investigate reproductive immunity.
• **Free radical attack** (*see* page 36) Research is being done on the vulnerability of embryos to free radical damage, and whether a good supply of antioxidants (*see* pages 15 and 20) via the developing placenta can prevent miscarriage in the first trimester.

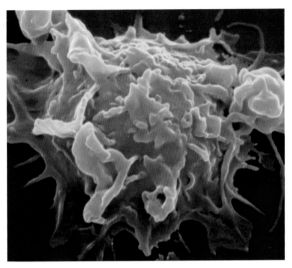

This natural killer cell is part of the body's immune system, and will aggressively attack rapidly growing or dividing cells.

Immunological disorders

The normal reaction of the body is to reject any "foreign" tissue, but when a woman becomes pregnant, alterations in her immune system prevent the destruction of the embryo. However, there are now thought to be immunity issues that can cause rejection. In some women, the immune system overreacts and attacks the developing embryo. Certain disorders of the blood can also prevent the embryo from developing.

The main antibodies implicated are:
• **Natural killer (NK) cells** These cells are present in all of us and they help fight infections. Occasionally, however, they can act aggressively and attack the embryo. Treatment is with a combination of drugs that may include aspirin, heparin, or immunoglobulins. The use of some of these drugs is controversial and the medical establishment is divided over their use.
• **Antiphospholipid antibodies** Phospholipids are normal cell components, some of which have gluelike properties that allow cells to stick together. During pregnancy, the blood becomes stickier and the risk of blood clotting increases. In the formation of the placenta, small cells fuse into

larger ones that are important for the supply of nutrients to the baby. Antiphospholipid antibodies (APLAs) cause damage to the inside of the placental blood vessels, leading to clotting and a reduction in blood flow and nutrient delivery. They can prevent implantation and affect the blood circulation between mother and embryo. Treatment of APLAs takes the form of anticoagulant (anti-clotting) medications—namely heparin and low-dose (baby) aspirin (under medical supervision).

• **Antinuclear antibodies (ANAs)** These antibodies thin the blood and can cause the placenta to become inflamed and weakened. Treatment is with corticosteroids. ANAs are also associated with diseases such as systemic lupus erythematosus, an autoimmune disorder that may affect several of the body's systems, and can lead to recurrent miscarriage, late pregnancy complications, and an increased risk of maternal thrombosis.

Balancing immunity

Since some of the drugs used in the treatment of implantation problems suppress the immune system, it is important to support treatment with a good diet. Eat plenty of fruit, vegetables, whole grains, and protein. Essential fatty acids (*see* page 21) balance the immune system and have been found to reduce irregular activity of NK cells. Avoid sugary foods, since sugar suppresses the immune system, and drink plenty of fluids.

Suppressing immunity can be balanced effectively with supplementation. A good prenatal vitamin and mineral supplement will ensure that you suffer no nutritional deficiencies as a result of the drugs you may be taking. In addition, a high-quality probiotic, such as a yogurt drink containing beneficial bacteria, will help maintain the population of these bacteria in the gut, which is important for a healthy immune system.

Finally, it is important to take care generally while you are taking these medications. Stress, overwork, fatigue, and illness will all compromise your immune system.

Free radicals and the embryo

It is thought that the embryo's need for oxygen varies at different stages of its development, rather than being constant. Early on, at the blastocyst stage, a high oxygen level is toxic, and studies show that the placenta develops in a low-oxygen environment as nutrients are transferred to the trophoblasts from the uterine lining. However, once the fetal circulation is fully established with the mother's, the fetus is exposed to oxygen and the harmful by-products of oxygen metabolism—free radicals (*see* page 15). Placental tissues contain low concentrations of antioxidant enzymes, and are therefore vulnerable to free radical attack. The fetus needs to start building up its own antioxidant circulation.

IF YOU ARE AT RISK

Most women will accept one miscarriage, but the more frequently it happens, the harder it is to accept. In time, they lose confidence in their body's ability to carry a pregnancy through.

Women who are at greater risk are those who have previously had a miscarriage, are over 35, smoke, are anorexic, drink a lot of alcohol, are exposed to radiation or environmental toxins, are suffering severe stress and anxiety, use cocaine, or have an underlying medical condition such as thyroid dysfunction or autoimmunity problems. I advise women who have had a miscarriage previously to stay close to home in the early stages of a subsequent pregnancy, and not to fly, have sex, or drink coffee. There is no hard evidence to support some of these links, but I think it is best to play safe.

As always, an approach that takes lifestyle factors and medical considerations into account is the best way forward. Preparing well for pregnancy and taking great care of yourself once you are pregnant will help reduce many of the risks. If you have already had a miscarriage or you are over 35, don't "just keep trying." It is important to get yourself checked by a specialist.

assisting fertility

More and more couples who have been having difficulty conceiving are opting for assisted reproductive technology. There are several options and combinations of treatments available, and your treatment will be adapted to your individual circumstances, your age, and the results of a variety of tests.

TIMED INTERCOURSE (TI)

If you have an irregular menstrual cycle, ovulation is difficult to predict. Ultrasound scans will be done at weekly intervals to determine when ovulation has occurred—this is known as follicular tracking. You and your partner can then have sexual intercourse at the appropriate time.

OVULATION INDUCTION (OI)

Ovulation induction, or ovarian stimulation, is a way of kick-starting ovulation to give you a chance of conceiving naturally. It can be used if you have irregular or absent periods due to an inadequate or imbalanced release of hormones, or if you are not ovulating because you have polycystic ovaries.

You'll be given a course of clomiphene citrate (in pill form) to be taken for two to five days each month, starting shortly after your cycle begins. This fools your system into thinking that estrogen levels are too low, which

stimulates the release of hormones that cause follicles to mature, ready for ovulation.

An injection of HCG (human chorionic gonadotropin) may also be given to encourage the final maturation of the follicle and the release of the egg. Intercourse or IUI (see below) will be timed for 36 to 40 hours after the injection.

INTRA-UTERINE INSEMINATION (IUI)

This is generally used when there is a problem with sperm motility and in some cases of unexplained infertility.

The aim is to place as many active sperm as possible as close as possible to the egg. A sample of washed sperm is injected directly into the uterus through the cervix. Drugs stimulate the follicles and induce ovulation. The procedure is carried out as close as possible to the expected time of ovulation (ideally within six hours), which is determined by a scan.

IVF AND ICSI

IVF (see page 38) involves fertilization taking place outside the uterus. It improves the odds that sperm can find and fertilize an egg because they don't have to negotiate the fallopian tube. If the sperm are weak and cannot fertilize the egg without further help, they may be injected into the egg by means of a procedure called intra-cytoplasmic sperm injection (ICSI).

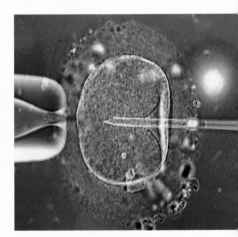

ICSI involves a single sperm being injected into the egg using a fine glass needle under a microscope.

undergoing in vitro fertilization

In vitro fertilization (IVF) involves an egg being removed from your body and fertilized in a laboratory under carefully controlled conditions.

PREPARING FOR IVF

I believe in preparing for IVF just as you would do for a natural pregnancy. There is research indicating that stress, weight, and even the time of year can all influence the success rate of IVF, so laying down good ground work, as we have discussed throughout Chapter 1, is vitally important. I also firmly believe in using supporting treatments during an IVF cycle.

Nutrition

Good nutrition helps support your body's ability to grow and nourish eggs, build up the lining of the uterus, heal after egg retrieval, and prepare for implantation.

• Egg quality will be one of your overriding concerns. Make sure you eat adequate protein. The best foods for amino acid balance are eggs, soy, meat, fish, beans, lentils, and quinoa.

• Take a good-quality multivitamin and mineral supplement to nourish your eggs.

• Essential fatty acids are vitally important, not least because most of us are deficient in them. If you are not already doing so, start taking a DHA supplement leading up to and during IVF treatment,.

• Drink at least two quarts (2 liters) of water (filtered or uncarbonated bottled) a day—in addition to other fluids such as herbal teas. This is important for cell formation and to ensure that the drugs get to where they need to go in the body.

Health

• If you have any longstanding complaints or health concerns, try to resolve them before you start IVF. Build up your energy reserves beforehand by getting lots of sleep, exercising, and eating well.

• You will have only minor surgery but you need to be able to repair quickly to receive the incoming embryos. Check that the multivitamin and mineral supplement you are taking contains zinc and take the homeopathic remedy Arnica 6c four times during the 24 hours before the procedure.

Lifestyle

• You give IVF a better chance if you're not overweight. If you need to, lose weight slowly and gradually, without depriving yourself of vital nutrients.

HOW IVF WORKS

Ten to twenty follicles are "cultivated" by means of hormone and other drug treatment. Further drugs are administered 36 hours before egg collection to release the eggs and mature them before they are extracted by a probe under general anesthetic. The fertilized eggs are placed in the uterus, which has been prepared hormonally to receive an embryo.

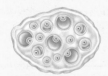

Day 12 of menstrual cycle Eggs mature, ready for collection

Day 13 Eggs are retrieved using a vaginal ultrasound or laparoscopy

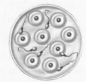

Day 14 IVF or ICSI method used to fertilize mature eggs

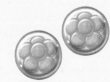

Day 15–18 Embryos loaded into catheter and inserted into the uterus

Likewise, if you are seriously underweight, gain weight sensibly.

• Avoid smoky atmospheres. The chemicals in cigarette smoke adversely affect the uterine lining.

• Avoid aerobic exercise. Your body needs rest as your hormonal system shuts down to prepare for IVF. Do gentle forms of exercise, such as walking, swimming, and yoga.

• Rest between 5 and 7pm—according to Traditional Chinese Medicine (TCM), reproductive function is governed by the kidneys and resting between these times is key to increasing their energy levels.

• Find a relaxation technique that suits you. Try meditation, yoga, or T'ai Chi.

• Use visualization (*see* page 67) to encourage a positive outcome —picture the eggs maturing, the uterine lining ripening, and the embryos implanting.

• Research shows that acupuncture may help relieve stress and balance the body, build up the uterine lining by improving pelvic blood flow, and grow follicles. After the eggs have been transferred to your uterus, it may encourage implantation and the maintenance of a pregnancy.

• Reflexology can be helpful in preparation for IVF, particularly on the parts of the foot corresponding to the pelvis and lymphatic system. Tell the practitioner you are planning a pregnancy.

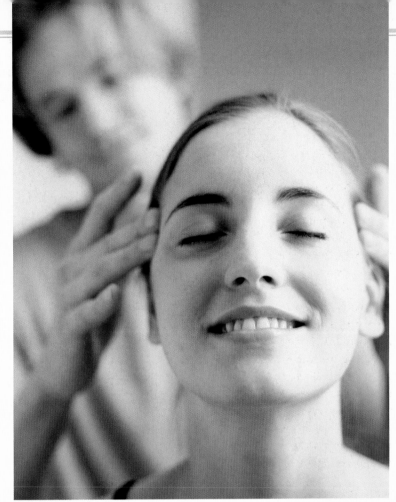

WAITING AND NURTURING

Once you have undergone all the IVF procedures, you have a couple of weeks to wait and see if an embryo implants and you become pregnant. You must nurture yourself during this time. Avoid caffeine, smoking, alcohol, and drugs; heavy lifting; strenuous exercise and housework; bouncing activities (such as horseback riding or aerobics); sun-bathing, Jacuzzis, saunas and hot tubs, and hot baths; swimming; sexual intercourse and orgasm. Visualize the embryos floating safely and preparing to embed.

Relaxation and stress relief are key to your preparation for IVF—find techniques that fit easily into your life.

You may feel emotionally wobbly at times as well as suffering physical symptoms such as sore breasts, slight spotting, mild shooting pains, and bloating. Concentrate on relaxation techniques and stress relief to help stimulate endorphins and the hormones that support the uterus, creating a nourishing environment for the embryo. Once you are back at work, try to take things easy and avoid stressful situations.

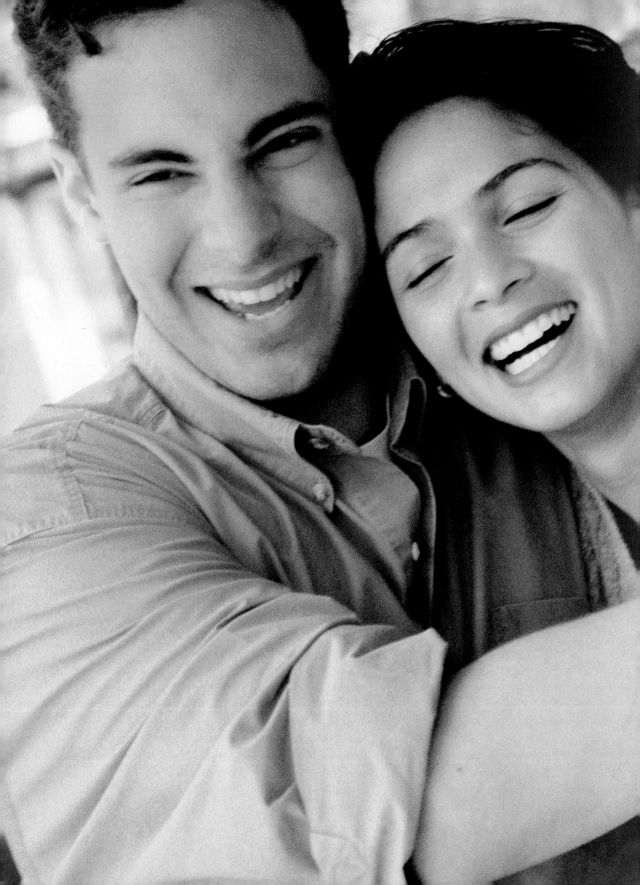

NOW THAT YOU'RE PREGNANT

This chapter starts with the discovery that you are expecting, then travels through the **three trimesters of pregnancy**. In each section, there is a detailed guide to what is happening to both you and your baby, with a **"windows of opportunity"** feature pinpointing chances to maximize your baby's healthy development. **Eating plans, exercise programs, and stress management techniques** are tailored to each stage of pregnancy, and features on **bonding** and **expecting more than one baby** appear throughout.

the first few weeks

I cannot emphasize enough the importance of the first trimester. During these early weeks, not only will the foundations be laid for the development of all your baby's organs, but also for a resilient pregnancy throughout.

MIXED EMOTIONS

Many women expect to be happy when they get a positive pregnancy test, but, often, anxiety seems to take over very quickly, especially if they've had an assisted fertility procedure. It can also be difficult if you have many demands on you at work while you get used to what's happening in your body, especially if you're experiencing symptoms such as nausea and vomiting or overwhelming fatigue.

We're bombarded with information about what's good and what's bad for us these days, so naturally many women have questions and concerns when they discover they are pregnant. And your first prenatal appointment may be weeks away.

GETTING OFF TO A GOOD START

Good implantation and the placenta's establishment of a sound "root system" of blood vessels in the womb lining (*see* page 56) will help prevent problems later in pregnancy, such as the fetus not growing, preeclampsia (*see* page 96), or premature labor (*see* pages 114–15). These problems are believed to have their origins in an inadequate foundation for the placenta, with free radical damage (*see* page 15) a contributory factor.

Pregnancy following IVF or miscarriage

If you've had a miscarriage previously or you've had IVF, you are bound to be more anxious. You'll be aware of every slight change in your body, from a twinge to an ache. You'll probably be running to the toilet every five minutes to see if there are any signs of bleeding. You may experience spotting, which is not uncommon with IVF, and therefore worry about miscarrying. Spotting is quite common and may mean that one of the embryos is coming away.

With an IVF baby, you will have more scans in the early stages of pregnancy to check that the embryo has embedded in the uterus (sometimes

---

IS YOUR PREGNANCY AT RISK?

If you've had a baby or been pregnant before and have had experiences that may put you at risk in subsequent pregnancies, you must inform anyone connected with your prenatal care and take even better care of yourself. This also applies to women with certain underlying health conditions.

Circumstances that are cause for extra care include:
- Previous ectopic pregnancy
- Recurrent miscarriage
- Termination with complications
- Preeclampsia
- History of blood disorders
- Excessive, prolonged bleeding

- Baby born with a congenital abnormality
- Baby who weighed more than 9lb (4kg) or less than 5lb 8oz (2.5kg) at birth
- Twins or other multiple pregnancy
- Diabetes
- Thyroid problems

it can float back into a fallopian tube, resulting in an ectopic pregnancy).

However, despite all the concerns, with each week that passes once you are pregnant, your chances of going to term get better and better. Don't read books or scour the internet if you are going to scare yourself even more: try to keep calm and think positively. And don't worry that you're not feeling the way you think you should be feeling. A variety of emotions is perfectly normal at this stage.

You may not feel like broadcasting your news from the rooftops. You and your partner may decide to confide only in family and very close friends until after 12 weeks, when you can be more confident that everything will be fine. If you've had a miscarriage before, you won't relax until you get beyond the point at which you miscarried last time. Once you've had your first routine scan and seen your baby's heartbeat, you're likely to be reassured and will probably start to be more optimistic about sharing your news.

PROGRAM FOR PREGNANCY

This starts the minute you get a positive pregnancy test. It's time to have another look at all the aspects of your health, diet, and lifestyle that you examined prior to embarking on a preconceptual care program (*see* pages 16–19, 22–9), but this time with the particular demands of each stage of your pregnancy in mind. Although it isn't very fashionable to say so, I recommend that women rest as much as they can during the first few months of pregnancy. I also advise that they drink no alcohol, because all alcohol is fetotoxic: it crosses the placenta and will directly affect the growing baby.

As soon as you discover you are pregnant you should exchange your preconception multivitamin and mineral supplement (*see* page 19) for one that is specially designed for pregnant women. Make sure it contains at least 400mcg of folic acid a day; if not, take a folic acid supplement separately (*see* page 59). Always check the dosage

of individual ingredients in your multivitamin and mineral supplement before taking any additional supplements.

Avoid caffeine, alcohol, tobacco, strenuous exercise and hot baths, saunas, or steam rooms. I also recommend that you avoid sexual intercourse during the first 12 weeks, although there is nothing to stop couples being sexually intimate in other ways. And I don't advise flying during the first trimester, especially long-haul.

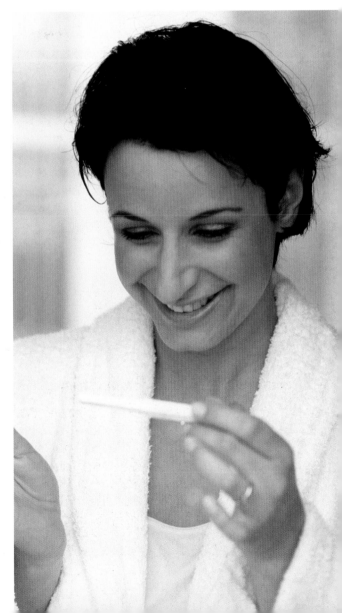

extraordinary pregnancies

Not every pregnancy arises as a result of careful planning, or involves a single embryo. In some cases, events take an unexpected course and when this happens you may find yourself drawing heavily on your physical and emotional reserves.

EXPECTING MORE THAN ONE

There are greater numbers of twin and triplet pregnancies now than ever before, largely because of assisted fertility techniques and because more women are having babies later in life. If you have a family history of twins, the news that you are carrying more than one baby won't come as such a surprise. But you will still have to adjust to the idea of nurturing and then caring for two (or more) tiny infants simultaneously. Multiple pregnancies are more at risk of complications, but you will be monitored carefully throughout. We will be looking at the special needs of your babies, trimester by trimester (*see* pages 68–9, 86–7, and 106–7).

Women who opt for assisted fertility techniques sometimes find themselves expecting twins, triplets, or even quads. This can present a huge dilemma if they are then faced with the difficult decision of whether or not to reduce the number of babies they are carrying. If this happens to you, you'll need to talk through the issues with your consultant. The decision will depend upon your health and how the pregnancy is progressing.

BABIES OUT OF THE BLUE

Many of the women I see are trying desperately to conceive and it seems amazing to me today that there can be any unexpected pregnancies. That's not to say that there aren't surprises. Sometimes, despite all sorts of complications, such as blocked tubes, high hormone levels, or a partner who has problem sperm, they find themselves pregnant.

The main reaction of women who fall pregnant unexpectedly

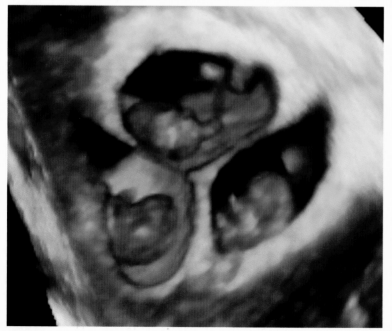

Multiple pregnancies have increased dramatically over recent years. Here three fetuses can be seen in utero.

is a feeling of being totally unprepared. Panic sets in that they have drunk too much wine, eaten too many processed foods or smoked too many cigarettes, and their baby may have suffered as a result. Reading the first chapter of this book may add to that panic. No one can reassure you totally. The best thing you can do is to make changes immediately. Cut out alcohol; if you smoke, stop; review your eating habits (*see* pages 16–19, 46–7, 60–1); and start taking multivitamin and mineral and folic acid supplements right away.

An unexpected pregnancy often brings with it emotional stress, too. What I would urge you to do is to keep calm and try to think ahead. Many of the women I see who have terminated an unexpected pregnancy in the past have emotional problems if they try to conceive later and find they have difficulties. Remember, there is always a way out.

Other concerns

If you find out that you are pregnant unexpectedly, you may worry about having been around children who have childhood diseases such as chickenpox, rubella, or mumps if you have not had the disease yourself or been immunized. If you do develop any symptoms in early pregnancy of diseases that can affect a fetus, get them checked

WILL TWINS BE IDENTICAL?

Identical, or monozygotic, twins are formed when one egg divides into two. Identical twins have the same DNA and are the same sex. They may share a placenta and an amniotic sac. Fraternal, or dizygotic, twins are formed when more than one egg is released and fertilized by different sperm. They have different combinations of genes like any other siblings. About two thirds of twins are fraternal. IVF accounts for the increasing number.

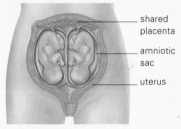

shared placenta
amniotic sac
uterus

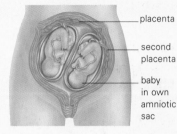

placenta
second placenta
baby in own amniotic sac

  one fertilized egg divides

 two separate eggs are fertilized

Identical twins are formed when one fertilized egg divides into two.

Nonidentical twins result from two eggs being fertilized by two sperm.

out by your physician or midwife and, in any case they should give you a blood test to check your immunity (*see* page 14). Discuss any medications you are taking, such as antibiotics. You may be concerned that you've eaten raw fish or meat recently, or you might have been dealing with cat litter and be worried about contracting toxoplasmosis. If you are in any doubt at all, talk to your doctor, who will arrange tests if need be.

DONOR EGGS AND SPERM

If you are unable to have your own child, or you or your partner risk passing on a genetic disorder, you may consider donor eggs or sperm. Despite careful screening, there will inevitably be many stresses and strains accompanying this decision. Couples worry about lots of issues, such as other people finding out; the potential inequality of only one partner being a biological parent; and whether they will feel differently about the baby when it is born.

Counseling is vitally important because of potential ethical, social, and legal problems; it will also help with the psychological and emotional implications. Above all, you and your partner should take time to mull over all the issues.

food rules

In the early days of pregnancy a lot of women feel that they're not eating as well as they were before they conceived. You may find you crave carbohydrates, even though you don't know why, and you may worry that you are going to gain too much weight.

HEALTHY TIPS

It takes time in the early days to establish just how much energy your body needs and how to control it. You need carbohydrates for energy so your body starts to crave them. Eating regularly will help.

Before we look at the specific requirements of your fetus in the first trimester (*see* pages 58–9), we need to establish the ground rules for your nutritional health throughout your pregnancy.

• Eat little and often to balance your blood-sugar levels. Mix protein with carbohydrate.

• Eat healthy snacks such as oatcakes and hummus, dried apricots, figs, cashews, live yogurt.

• Avoid sugary, refined, and processed foods. Use organic honey or jams made without extra sugar and eat organic chocolate when you need a "fix."

• Reduce the amount of saturated fat in your diet. Drink low-fat milk and trim the fat off meat and the skin off chicken.

• Choose organic food wherever possible.

• Eat good-quality, lean protein—fish (not farmed), chicken, legumes, and occasionally tofu.

• Choose healthy fish options. Eat fresh white fish and organic oily fish, such as salmon, trout, herring, mackerel, and haddock.

• Reduce your intake of high-fat dairy products.

• Reduce wheat, which some people find difficult to digest. It also binds to valuable minerals such as iron and zinc, preventing absorption.

• Drink herbal teas and coffee substitutes such as dandelion root tea.

• Avoid hydrogenated fats, which are found in margarines and many cookies and crackers. These interfere with the production of essential fats.

• Avoid salt. Eat more potassium-rich foods (fruits and vegetables) if you want to reduce symptoms of fluid retention. Garlic, herbs, spices, lemon juice and black pepper all enhance flavor and contain

VEGETARIAN PREGNANCY

If you are vegetarian, it is very important to make sure you maintain a balanced, healthy diet during pregnancy. You can obtain your protein, vitamin B_{12}, calcium, and iron from a variety of sources:

● nuts such as almonds, Brazil nuts, cashews, and nut butter

● legumes such as chickpeas (including

hummus), lentils, peas, and beans (including baked beans)

● seeds such as sesame, sunflower, and pumpkin

● dairy products, particularly low-fat ones such as yogurt and cottage cheese

● free-range organic eggs

● soy products such as soy milk, soy burgers and sausages, tofu

If you follow a vegan diet, combine plant proteins carefully to make sure you get enough essential amino acids. For example, add a portion of nuts or peas to a rice dish. Eat plenty of green beans, cereals, and dried fruits such as prunes, apricots, or raisins to maintain your iron intake. Consult your doctor about taking supplements.

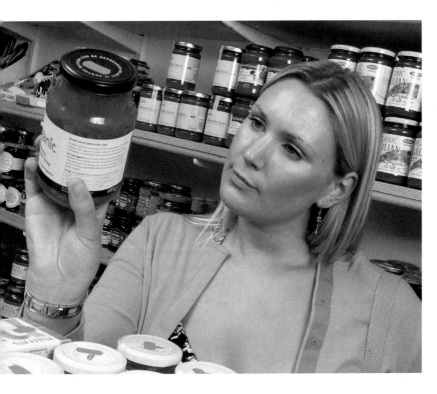

"avoid food additives wherever possible. Get used to reading labels."

antioxidant, anti-inflammatory plant compounds.
• Increase the amount of fiber in your diet by eating flaxseeds, oats and oat bran, fruit, and vegetables.
• Eat a wide variety of colored fruits and vegetables, such as mangoes and red peppers.
• Drink at least 3.5 pints (1.5 liters) of filtered water a day.
• Avoid food additives whenever possible. Learn how to read food labels.

Buying and preparing food

There are many health food stores where you can buy the foods I have recommended. But local stores and supermarkets are often good enough, and many carry a wide range of organic foods as well as wheat and dairy alternatives.

Whenever possible, avoid foods wrapped in plastic by buying loose fruit and vegetables and meat from the butcher's counter. Store foods in glass containers rather than plastic ones and don't use plastic wrap or aluminum foil.

Wash fruit and vegetables before you prepare them and don't eat uncooked or raw meats, which might have been infected with toxoplasmosis. This is a parasitic infection carried in cat feces and can have serious effects on the fetus.

Eat as much local and seasonal fruit and vegetables as possible. Try not to cook your food in aluminum or unlined copper pots and pans. Avoid microwaving in order to limit your exposure to radiation and your intake of damaging free radicals. Valuable fat-soluble vitamins are also destroyed in the microwave.

As far as cooking methods are concerned, steaming, sweating, baking, and stir-frying preserve nutrients better. Don't overcook vegetables—five minutes' steaming for green vegetables is plenty. Use only a little cold-pressed, extra virgin, organic olive oil. High temperatures damage most vegetable oils; olive oil is the most stable. Finally, avoid barbequeing —cooking and charring foods at high temperatures causes the formation of carcinogenic agents.

what's safe, what's not

When you are first pregnant, you'll probably have concerns about what you should and shouldn't avoid. Steering clear of the long lists of things that you have heard can be hazardous in pregnancy may seem daunting at the beginning; this guide will help you get into the habit of knowing what's safe and what's not.

FOODS TO AVOID

Early in pregnancy you may worry when you realize that you've eaten something on the "foods to avoid" list. This is easily done, but don't panic. If you follow the basic rules of hygiene—washing everything, avoiding contamination between raw and prepared food, defrosting and reheating food

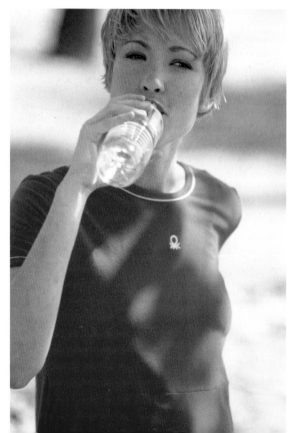

thoroughly, and avoiding food past its sell-by date—you are unlikely to contract an infection.

There are some foods that are best forgotten about for the next nine months.

• Those that are more likely to contain pathogenic bacteria such as listeria or salmonella. These tend to be unpasteurized foods such as soft cheeses (brie, camembert) and blue cheeses; patés; chilled foods that have not been stored well; bagged salads; dishes containing raw or undercooked fish and shellfish, raw meat, and raw eggs.

• Those containing high levels of environmental pollutants, such as large predatory fish (tuna, swordfish, or shark), which are high in mercury, or chemicals used in food production, such as farmed salmon, or intensively grown fruit and vegetables.

• Those containing naturally toxic substances, such as green potatoes, which contain glycoalkaloids, or those in which toxins form during processing, such as alcohol, which produces acetaldehyde as it is metabolized by your body.

• Those that cause allergy, such as peanuts, if there is a family history on your or your partner's side.

• Liver, which may have too much vitamin A, a vitamin that has been linked to fetal abnormality in pregnancy. Liver also processes toxins.

• Caffeine, which has been linked to miscarriage.

Drink filtered or bottled water, since they do not contain the high levels of chlorine and fluoride found in tap water.

ENVIRONMENTAL CHECKLIST

To ensure that your surroundings are safe especially during early pregnancy:

● Minimize your exposure to environmental chemicals: don't decide to lay new carpets, or strip off old paint.

● Avoid strong household cleaning products: many stores stock milder alternatives, or you can use alternatives such as vinegar or lemon juice.

● Keep car windows closed when you are in heavy traffic.

● Minimize time spent near sources of electromagnetic radiation.

● Don't use artificial air fresheners, artificially scented candles, or potpourri mixes. Be aware of chemicals in cleansers, deodorants, and other beauty products (see pages 28–9).

● Avoid perfumes and aftershave lotions because many contain phthalates. Try flower waters instead.

● If you have a cat, avoid contact with its litter tray to minimize the risk of catching toxoplasmosis (see page 47).

● Avoid cigarette smoke.

● Drink filtered or bottled water.

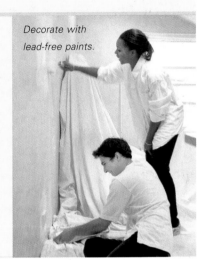

Decorate with lead-free paints.

In addition, avoid where possible packaged low-fat products—they're full of chemicals and additives; don't eat highly processed foods—they're laden with fats and salt; and eat vegetables and fruit in as close to their natural state as possible.

DRUGS IN PREGNANCY

Many women are concerned about which medicines they can use during pregnancy. I would say take as few prescription or nonprescription drugs as possible, unless absolutely necessary. Those to avoid include acne medication (accutane is linked to miscarriage and birth defects); certain antibiotics (tetracyclines, streptomycin, sulfonamides); antimalarials (linked to embryonic abnormalities); and some laxatives. Other drugs, such as some antihistamines, some cold and flu remedies (they contain caffeine), some laxatives, aspirin, steroids and diuretics are contraindicated in pregnancy, so always consult your doctor before you self-treat a complaint.

Certain herbal remedies are unsuitable for use during pregnancy because of their potentially adverse effects on the fetus, so if you are considering using any of these always consult a qualified herbalist first.

ADDITIVE AWARENESS

Everybody suspects that colorings and preservatives added to foods do nothing for our health, but do you know just how bad they are?

● **Monosodium glutamate/E621.** Added to savory processed foods. Linked to nerve cell damage in the brain, DNA damage, and fetal abnormalities in animals.

● **Aspartame/E951.** Sweetener. May cause damage to the developing brain (it crosses the placenta).

● **Acesulfame K/E950.** Sweetener. Linked to blood sugar imbalances and raised cholesterol levels.

● **Saccharine/E954.** Sweetener. Causes DNA damage and congenital abnormalities in animals and may result in blood-sugar imbalance.

● **Sodium benzoate/E211.** Preservative used in soft drinks, baked goods, and candies. Suspected to be neurotoxic, carcinogenic, and to cause fetal abnormalities.

● **Sulfur dioxide/E220.** Preservative used in soft drinks, dried fruits, potato products. Responsible for DNA damage and fetal abnormalities in animals.

● **Quinoline yellow/E104.** Coloring used in soft drinks, desserts, and sauces. Affects reproduction in animals.

● **Sunset yellow/E110.** Coloring used in snacks, drinks, ice cream, and sweets. Linked to DNA damage.

the older mother

Years ago, when I was doing midwifery, anyone over 26 was considered to be an older mother. Now, it's more like 37 and many of my clients are in their late 30s or early 40s. In the UK in the past 10 years, the number of women over 40 having babies has doubled and is now more than 2 percent.

MATURE MOTHERHOOD

Many women delay motherhood through choice, while others have problems conceiving or have one or more miscarriages so they have delay forced upon them. Older women may have fewer financial worries and be in more stable relationships, but their anxiety levels are likely to be high during pregnancy and labor, especially if they've had IVF. This may, of course, reflect the fact that the older you are, the more you know.

The advantages

Women today are fitter and healthier; there are highly technical procedures to help them conceive; and their lifestyles are much improved since their grandmothers were having babies. So don't listen to too many gloomy statistics about older mothers and the possible complications in pregnancy. There is plenty of evidence to show that a healthy woman in her 40s can have a healthy baby.

One advantage of being older is that you will feel more confident about making choices, such as whether to have tests or not. You may also be more ready to have a child because you already have a sense of fulfilment in other areas of life. Research shows that older mothers are more likely to make time to enjoy their children. They are also more likely to breastfeed and their children may perform better at school.

Lifestyle adjustments

If you are older, you may feel more tired during pregnancy than your younger counterparts, and you'll need longer to adjust to the changes going on in your body. It's important during the first trimester to rest frequently. You are more likely to be a professional, and you will have to consciously build time into your routine for rest. You may well have to go to bed early most nights. You may also have to give up work earlier than usual, at about 34 weeks. Nutritionally, it's

vitally important that you pay attention to balancing blood-sugar levels (*see* page 61).

The risk of complications

Women over 35 are at greater risk of miscarrying, of developing high blood pressure or pregnancy-induced diabetes, as well as some of the late-pregnancy problems. In many cases, however, modern obstetrics can monitor and treat these problems, and, as an older mother-to-be, you're more likely to be under consultant care.

As older women are well aware, the risk of Down syndrome increases from 1 in 400 at aged 35 to 1 in 109 at 40 and 1 in 32 beyond 45. Other rarer chromosomal abnormalities such as Patau syndrome and Edward syndrome are also more likely with increasing age.

Increased monitoring

Mothers over 35 are likely to have more prenatal tests and scans than younger women, but

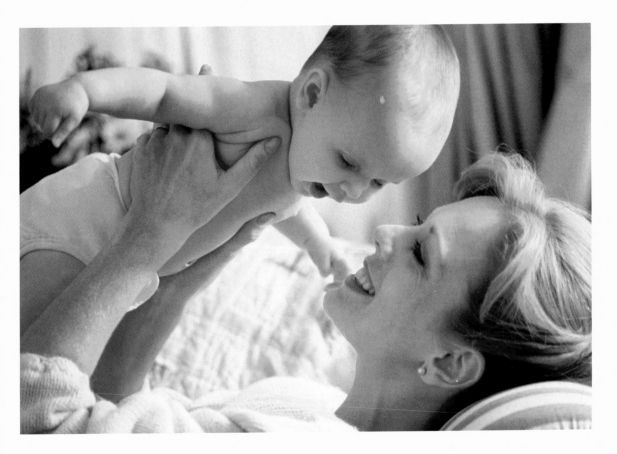

monitoring can be reassuring. Where there are no tangible medical complications, the risks of childbirth are no greater for older women.

Multiple births

The incidence of multiple birth increases with age, more so for nonidentical twins. According to research carried out at the National Institute of Child Health and Human Development, twins and triplets born to older women are as healthy as those born to younger mothers.

Statistics show that older women are more likely to have low birthweight babies (those that weigh less than 5lb 8oz/2.5kg). However, a closer look at these figures suggests that the difference is probably related to the increased incidence of multiple births in older women, so it is important when dealing with statistics to make sure you get a full picture of the information available.

Health beyond birth

According to a study in the *British Medical Journal*, there is an increased risk of the first babies of older mothers developing diabetes. The

In the UK, the number of women over 40 having babies has doubled in the past 10 years.

mother's age at delivery seems to be strongly related to the risk of type 1 (insulin-dependent) diabetes, a woman in her mid 40s being more than three times more likely to have a child who develops diabetes than a woman who is 20. This emphasizes the importance of maintaining a good blood-sugar balance throughout your pregnancy, not only from the point of view of sustaining you, but also ensuring your baby's health in the future.

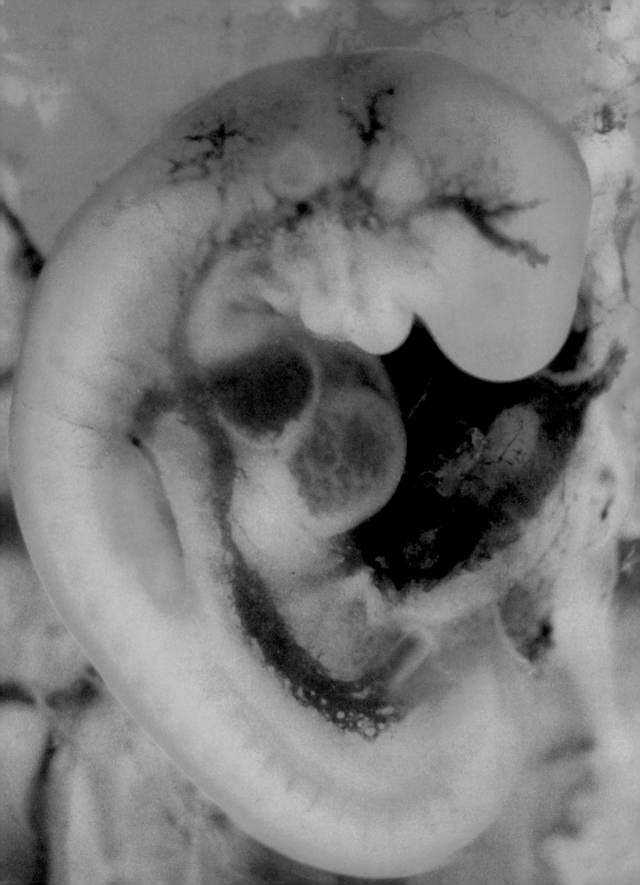

FIRST TRIMESTER
what's happening?

Some women know they're pregnant before they've even missed a period. For others, in the week leading up to what would have been their period, their breasts feel tender, they'll be tired and perhaps unusually sensitive to scents. Others won't get any signs at all, and they might not suspect they're pregnant for weeks.

LAYING FOUNDATIONS

Just a week or so after embryo implantation, rapid changes take place daily as the foundations of your pregnancy are laid down. Some of the cells in the developing placenta produce the hormone human chorionic gonadotropin (HCG), which signals to the ovaries and pituitary gland that you're pregnant. Progesterone produced by the corpus luteum has already raised your body temperature ready to warm and nurture the embryo.

CELL DIFFERENTIATION

Cell division occurs in the blastocyst, distinguishing placental cells from embryonic cells. At the same time, each individual cell is directed so that it has a specific function, such as a liver cell or a heart cell. Once it is "programmed" it cannot change into another type of cell. Within the embryonic cell cluster, a disk forms, which in turn develops three layers. The outermost layer becomes the brain, spinal cord, nerves, parts of the eyes and ears, skin, hair, nails, and tooth enamel. The cells in the middle layer develop into the skeleton, heart and other muscles, cartilage and connective tissue, blood cells and vessels, lymph cells and vessels, reproductive organs,

At five weeks, the 2mm-long embryo already has a rudimentary head curved over its bulging heart.

kidneys, and many glands. The inner layer forms the digestive system, mucous membranes, respiratory system, bladder, and urinary tract.

At day 15 after conception, nerve cells begin to form the brain and spinal column, and the brain sparks into action. Your blood volume increases to cope with the extra demand for oxygen.

KEY WEEK: 5 (3 WEEKS AFTER CONCEPTION)

In this critical week of rapid development, the embryo is very sensitive to potential damage. Organ formation begins in earnest, even though the embryo at this point would fit on the head of a nail. The embryo folds in on itself and forms a long tube. The top will form the head and the bottom the "tail."

COUNTING WEEKS IN PREGNANCY

You will be pregnant for about 38 weeks (266 days) from the moment of fertilization. This is obviously difficult to pinpoint, so your due date is calculated from the first day of your last period, which is usually about two weeks before fertilization takes place, making pregnancy 40 weeks long. So, what is in fact the third week of the embryo's development is called week five of the 40-week pregnancy, and so on. The first trimester is weeks 1–13, the second, weeks 14–28, and the third, weeks 29–40.

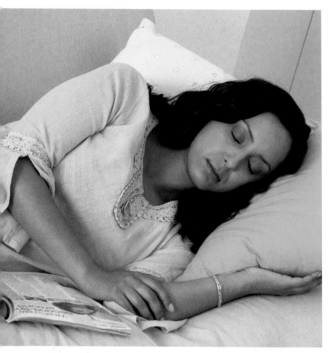

The heart

For the embryo to develop, it needs oxygen and nutrients circulating within it, so it is essential that the heart starts to pump blood as soon as possible. At the beginning of week five of pregnancy, the newly formed muscle suddenly contracts: one cell "beats," which triggers a domino reaction, and within a couple of days all the heart cells are beating as one. By week 11, the fetal heart will have developed chambers and valves.

The spinal cord

A long thickening forms in the area where the backbone and spinal cord will be, known as the neural plate. By the end of week six, the folds fuse around the groove, forming the neural tube. Groups of cells grow around the lower neural tube until they meet and fuse at the back, enclosing the developing spinal cord in a series of rings that eventually become the protective bony spinal column.

The brain

The brain develops from a bulge at one end of the neural tube. Folds and hollows form as nerve cells join forces and different areas of the brain take on the different functions of the forebrain, midbrain,

"early pregnancy symptoms include fatigue and nausea"

HOW YOUR BODY IS CHANGING

Your metabolism speeds up as all the organ systems in your body are adapting to the increasing demands placed upon them by your pregnancy. Your metabolic rate will increase by as much as 10–25 percent to allow the production of sufficient oxygen to reach all the tissues of all the organs.

To get it there, the amount of blood being pumped through the heart must increase—by 40–50 percent by the end of your pregnancy. (The actual amount varies according to the size of the woman, how many pregnancies she's had, and how many babies she's carrying.) This process takes place gradually: the watery component of blood, called plasma, starts to increase during the first six weeks of pregnancy to fill newly formed blood vessels in the placenta and other growing organs.

You might feel as though you need to empty your bladder more often than usual because the blood supply to the kidneys increases by about 30 percent, resulting in more blood being filtered and therefore more urine to eliminate. In addition, the enlarging uterus presses on the bladder. You may be more sensitive to smells and crave certain foods. You may not be able to tolerate tastes such as coffee, and you may develop a metallic taste in your mouth. Other early pregnancy symptoms include nausea, fatigue, breast tenderness, and heightened emotions.

and hindbrain. Once this happens, the basic structure of the fetal nervous system is in place. Very small hollows that will be the eyes and mouth are discernible.

By the time all this has happened, your pregnancy will just about have been confirmed.

WEEKS 6–10 (4–8 AFTER CONCEPTION)

The embryo continues to develop rapidly, tripling in size in seven days. It is shaped like a kidney bean. On either side of the spinal column, there are now vertebrae developing, and from between these, nerve cells radiate in an increasingly complex nervous system that reaches every part of the body. This network of nerves has two very important functions: it transmits to all muscles, telling them when to contract; and it passes information to the brain about the stimuli the nerves can register: sensations such as heat, pain, or pressure.

Blood vessels now extend into the head and around the body, and the heart is pumping blood throughout the circulatory system. Arm and leg buds become visible. Gradually the embryo starts to resemble a miniature human being.

The face

A human face is now beginning to build around the mouth. The lower jaw is the first to form at five weeks' gestation, then the upper jaw forms and the two fuse in the sixth week. Failure of this to happen will cause a cleft lip or cleft palate.

An embryo's head is very large in relation to the rest of its body. When it is born, its head will still make up a quarter of its total length, and only by puberty will the body assume its adult proportions.

Many of the fetal organs are now functioning—the kidneys are producing urine and the stomach produces gastric juices—and the embryo can move spontaneously. Movement is particularly important because it stimulates the growth of muscles and the development of joints.

By the end of the eighth week of gestation, the embryo has become a fetus. Up to this point, it has been dependent on the yolk sac (a balloonlike structure attached to the embryo by a stalk) for nutrients. The yolk sac now dissolves away and nutrients are supplied via the placenta, which now has more than 200 different cells (*see* pages 56–7).

WEEK 13 (11 WEEKS AFTER CONCEPTION)

By week 13, all your baby's vital body organs are in place and the fetus resembles a human being: eyelids are distinguishable on the face; brain and muscles coordinate; joints work; toes curl and fingers and toes have nails; the fetus can swallow.

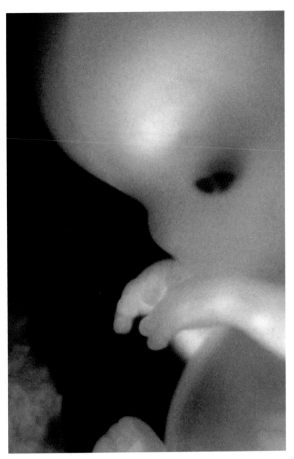

A fetus at 10 weeks: the eyes have now migrated from the sides of the head and the forehead is high and bulging.

the vital link

Revered by ancient civilizations and some cultures today, the placenta is an amazing organ. It is much more than a fetal supply line, in that it provides the foundation for your entire pregnancy. It could be described as a joint venture between you and your baby, in which an extraordinary exchange process takes place.

THE TREE OF LIFE

The ideal environment for the placenta to flourish is a thick, spongelike uterine lining that is alkaline. After implantation, the blastocyst's placental cells spread into the lining. The developing placenta begins to resemble a tree with a root system. The "roots" are in fact chorionic villi, fingerlike projections that extend from the membrane (the chorion) that surrounds the embryo from the time of implantation. Some roots are superficial while others embed deep into the uterine wall to access the mother's blood supply. Through them oxygen, nutrients, and waste are exchanged without the mother's and embryo's blood supplies mixing.

Between the placenta and the embryo runs the umbilical cord, which consists of a large vein carrying oxygenated blood from the placenta and two small arteries carrying waste products and deoxygenated blood back to the mother from the fetus.

Functions of the placenta

Uniquely formed from two individuals, each with a different genetic make-up, the placenta has a fetal component and a maternal component. It acts as a fetal lung and a fetal kidney, absorbing oxygen from and passing waste products out into the mother's bloodstream.

It also acts as a fetal digestive system. Every pulse of the mother's blood brings a varying supply of nutrients. Your baby's growth depends upon the quality of the nutritional service you supply and the size and efficiency of the placenta. The placenta actually grows faster than the baby during the second trimester. The larger the placenta grows, the more food your baby gets.

The placenta also acts as a barrier preventing the passage of toxins to the fetus. Unfortunately, however, it cannot prevent all harmful substances from getting through (*see* box on facing page).

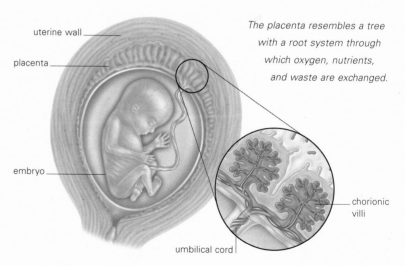

uterine wall

placenta

embryo

umbilical cord

chorionic villi

The placenta resembles a tree with a root system through which oxygen, nutrients, and waste are exchanged.

A hormone producer

One of the placenta's lesser-known but equally important functions is as a producer of hormones. In the beginning, its production of human chorionic gonadotropin (HCG) triggers the production of other pregnancy hormones. By the seventh or eighth week of pregnancy it is producing estrogen and progesterone to maintain the uterus.

The placenta also releases human placental lactogen (HPL), which stimulates milk glands in the breasts to be ready for breastfeeding. Ultimately, it starts the hormonal "conversation" between the fetus and the placenta that triggers labor.

FETAL SURVIVAL

There is only so much oxygen or energy the placenta can supply. Being an important organ, it consumes a lot of oxygen and glucose itself—in fact, about half of the amount provided by you. The survival of the fetus depends upon a healthy, thriving placenta so it is top of the list of priorities when it comes to maternal supplies.

If the fetus becomes short of oxygen, blood flow is diverted from less important functions in order to support the most vital organs under development, the brain and the heart. If oxygen supplies are not restored, then ultimately the placenta will fail and the fetus will stop growing. If supplies of glucose or important nutrients are similarly restricted, there will be a corresponding slowing of the growth of the fetus.

In later pregnancy, there may be competition between you and your baby for nutritional supplies: you need to build up your energy reserves to get ready for labor, while the placenta has to nourish a baby that is by now much larger and therefore has increasing nutritional demands. If this is the case, your needs will take priority over those of your baby.

Problems with placental function are often responsible for risks to the pregnancy near to term (*see* pages 96–9).

FOODS TO FEED THE PLACENTA

The key foods for the maintenance of optimum placental function are antioxidants and detoxifiers. Antioxidant foods (*see* page 61) or supplements providing coenzyme Q10, vitamins C and E, or garlic (which is also good for blood circulation and has antibiotic properties) are advisable. The enzyme glutathione is a particularly good antioxidant and detoxifier for placental health. It protects against damage by pollutants and is important for cell differentiation and proliferation in the developing embryo. Good food sources are asparagus, broccoli, avocado, and spinach.

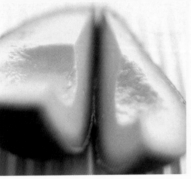

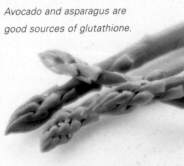

Avocado and asparagus are good sources of glutathione.

TERATOGENS

Teratogens are substances that cross the placental barrier, harming the embryo or fetus, sometimes causing birth defects. They include:

● drugs—medications, narcotics (morphine, opium), sedatives, analgesics, tranquilizers, antidepressants, nicotine, alcohol, marijuana, cocaine

● chemicals—heavy metals and environmental pollutants (lead, PCBs, dioxins)

● radiation (including X-rays)

● some maternal diseases caused by bacteria and viruses

● rubella

● toxoplasmosis (*see* page 47)

● sexually transmitted infections.

windows of opportunity
nutrition for growth

Between the third and eighth weeks of pregnancy the embryo undergoes astonishing physical changes. There is some fascinating research available about how nutrition and other factors influence your baby's development.

PROGRAMMED DEVELOPMENT

Research carried out by Professor Barker at the University of Southampton reveals how each fetal organ has a particular window of opportunity to grow. Whatever nutrients are needed for that to happen must be available precisely when they are required if that organ is to reach its full potential. If growth of the organ is limited at this critical time, it doesn't catch up afterward.

Now that you are pregnant, you need nutrient-rich food. Your body will become more efficient at absorbing nutrients as long as they are available. In particular, it will absorb key nutrients that the baby needs, such as calcium. The effects of poor nutrition during the first trimester are reduced birthweight, reduced head circumference, less than optimum brain development, and an increased risk of high blood pressure in later life.

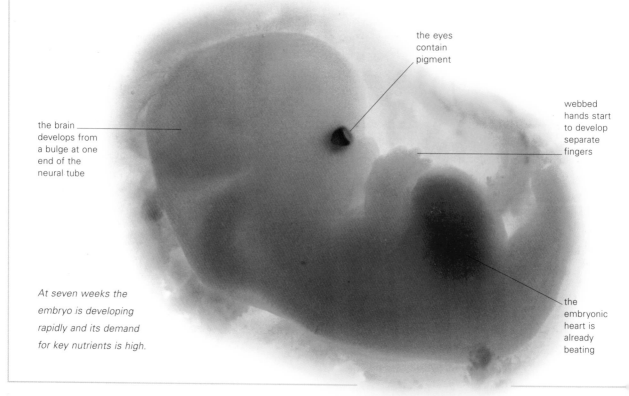

the eyes contain pigment

webbed hands start to develop separate fingers

the brain develops from a bulge at one end of the neural tube

the embryonic heart is already beating

At seven weeks the embryo is developing rapidly and its demand for key nutrients is high.

STAPLES FOR GROWTH

Ideally, a baby does not depend on how much its mother eats each day; it draws on her reserves. But for women who are undernourished when they conceive, the food they consume during pregnancy is of even greater significance.

Proteins consist of amino acids, which are vital for making hormones and for the repair and generation of new tissue for you and your baby. Protein intakes at the beginning of pregnancy correlate to the size of your baby at birth. Proteins also carry hormones, nutrients, and messages around the body.

Research is showing that nutrition affects the hormones that control a baby's growth, the most important of which is insulin. When a mother is undernourished the baby responds by reducing the amount of insulin it produces and slows its growth.

FOLIC ACID AND NTDS

The brain and spinal cord develop from an embryonic structure called the neural tube. This begins as a tiny ribbon of tissue that folds inward to form a tube by the 28th day after fertilization. When the neural tube does not close completely, defects in the brain and spinal cord may occur. Some 300,000 babies are born with neural tube defects (NTDs) in the world every year, while other affected pregnancies end in miscarriage or stillbirth. The most common NTDs are spina bifida and anencephaly (absence of a brain).

Exactly how folic acid prevents NTDs is not fully understood. Research suggests that it corrects a nutritional deficiency and, in some cases, helps people compensate for inborn errors in how the body processes folate. Folic acid aids the production of additional blood cells and is crucial in supporting the rapid growth of both placenta and fetus. Deficiency is also linked to premature birth and low birthweight, pregnancy-related high blood pressure, and, because it will limit the production of normal red blood cells, anemia.

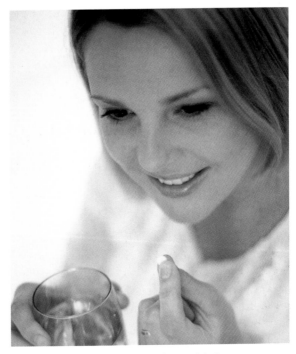

Taking a folic acid supplement before and during pregnancy helps reduce the incidence of neural tube defects.

BRAIN FOOD

Your baby's most complex organ, its brain, begins to develop as early as 18 days after conception (*see* page 54). The vital essential fatty acids needed must come from you since the fetus cannot manufacture its own (*see* page 21). If you do not have enough, the fetus will substitute inferior fatty acids, which may have long-term effects on its brain and nervous system.

Choline and iodine are also critical for brain development at this stage. Choline is needed for the manufacture of cell membranes and for cell division; is used by nerve cells; and, according to animal studies, is linked to the memory and learning centers of the brain. A balanced diet will usually deliver enough choline. Brain development will be stunted in the first trimester if the maternal supply of thyroid hormone is insufficient, and iodine is important for synthesis of this hormone (*see* pages 134–6 for sources of essential fats, choline, and iodine).

good eating plan

It takes a while when you are first pregnant to adjust to what
and when to eat as you get used to the demands placed upon
your body by the baby. Many women are shocked by how hungry
they feel. Others feel sick and can't bear the thought of food.
Try to eat something for breakfast no matter how bad you feel.

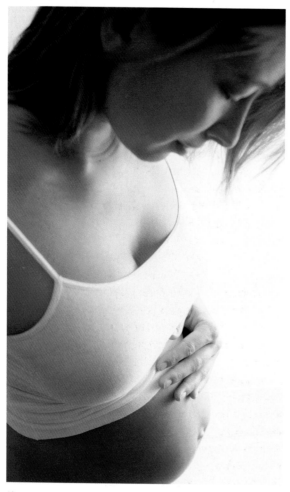

*If you stay within the recommended boundaries of weight
gain, you will ensure optimum health for your baby.*

GOOD BABY CARBS

Every woman enters pregnancy with different
nutritional needs, but balancing blood sugar is
vitally important for everyone. Your metabolism
will function properly, you will have more energy,
and you won't crave sweet, refined foods.

We have already looked at the basic guidelines
for eating to balance your blood-sugar levels (*see*
page 16); among the key things to remember are
to eat regularly. You can snack, but choose the
right snacks (*see* pages 46–7). And remember, if
you experience cravings, just a little of what you
want will usually be enough to satisfy the craving.

You need to eat "good baby carbs" so that your
baby receives a steady supply of glucose and can
grow at a steady rate. If the baby doesn't know
where the next meal is coming from, its body will go
into "shut down mode" in order to conserve energy.

Always mix protein and carbohydrate in a meal
to prolong the digestive process so that glucose is
released slowly. Good recipes that combine proteins
and carbs in proportion, often using only a little
animal protein, are found in Middle Eastern and
Asian cooking, where rice, beans, chickpeas, nuts,
and fruits are mixed with lamb, chicken, and fish.
Include peas and beans in your diet—they're a
ready-made mixture of protein and carbohydrate.

Try to eat your evening meal before seven o'clock.
If you get hungry later, have a snack, such as a
yogurt and banana with some seeds, before going

to bed. This will help increase levels of a sleep-inducing brain chemical called tryptophan, and prevent insomnia due to falling blood sugar in the night. The Chinese believe the stomach rests between seven and nine in the evening, and digestive problems, malabsorption of nutrients, and sleeplessness may be the result of eating late.

Blood sugar and the glycemic index

The glycemic index (GI) was originally devised to help people suffering from diabetes to control their blood-sugar levels. Operating on a scale of 1–100, it is based on how quickly a food is digested, metabolized, and released into the blood stream as glucose. It is useful for general health purposes too: foods that have a low or moderate GI ranking make us feel fuller for longer and encourage stable blood sugar.

Glucose is ranked 100 because it is absorbed most quickly, providing fast-release, short-term energy. Pure sugar products are best avoided altogether, or otherwise mixed with a little protein or fat, which slows down the process of glucose release. Avoid completely refined and processed foods with added sugars and sweeteners. How foods are cooked affects their GI ranking; for example, boiled potatoes are medium but mashed and baked potatoes are high; standard white rice is high while basmati is medium.

Foods with a low GI ranking include those that are higher in soluble fiber, such as most fruits and vegetables, wholegrains such as oats, and legumes. You should eat as many of these slow-release foods as possible. (For a fuller guide to the GI rating of different foods *see* page 137.)

FIRST TRIMESTER NUTRIENTS

Pregnant women need up to 60g of protein a day, so remember to eat a variety of protein foods to get a balance of all the amino acids. Antioxidant foods are vitally important in the body's fight against free radicals (*see* page 15). Eat plenty of fruit and vegetables containing carotenoids: these are a safe source of vitamin A, which is important for vision as well as cell division and differentiation. Selenium is an antioxidant trace mineral important to the immune system. Certain B vitamins are needed at this stage for the development of the baby's brain and nervous system. Choline and iodine are important for brain development, as is the essential fatty acid DHA. For food sources of all these nutrients *see* pages 134–7.

WEIGHT WATCH

Pregnant women frequently ask me "How much should I weigh?" or "How much weight should I put on?" Pregnancy gets blamed by some for excessive weight gain and lack of fitness. Others are convinced the weight gained is somehow different and will be impossible to shift after the birth. But if you gain the recommended amount of weight, you should have no problem losing it afterward.

That amount is 25–35lb (11–16kg). If your BMI (*see* page 23) is within the normal range, you should gain about 3½lb (1.5kg) in the first three months or so of pregnancy and then about 1lb (450g) a week after that. If you are underweight, you should gain 5lb (2.25kg) in the first three months and then slightly more than 1lb (450g) a week, giving a total weight gain of 28–40lb (13–18kg). If you are overweight, you should gain 2lb (900g) in the first three months, then about two thirds of a pound (300g) thereafter (total 15–25lb/7–11kg). If you are expecting twins, you can expect an overall weight gain of about 35–45lb (16–20kg).

For the fitness- and diet-obsessed, pregnancy presents the ultimate test of body control. Some women restrict their food intakes at this time, but while your baby can draw on your fat stores and thus get the calories it needs, it will not get the essential nutrients, which must be supplied on a daily basis.

Remember, your baby's birthweight is the single most important indicator of its future health.

looking at lifestyle

I believe the early weeks of pregnancy are extremely important: your baby is growing rapidly and using up a lot of energy. Follow your natural instincts—rest whenever you feel the need and take good care of yourself.

LIFESTYLE CHECKLIST

Following a few general rules can help you cope with the early stages of pregnancy, keeping both you and the growing fetus in good health.
• Have lots of early nights. Never underestimate the power of sleep to regenerate the body and build up your energy reserves.
• Avoid all aerobic exercise unless you've already attained a certain fitness level (*see* below).
• Don't embark on a long trip. There is no evidence that this is risky, but it can cause deep-vein thrombosis, whereby blood supply to the legs is reduced.
• Avoid hot baths. Heat can be damaging to the fetus, so have warm baths or showers instead.

EXERCISE IN EARLY PREGNANCY

There are many benefits of regular exercise in pregnancy for both mother and baby. It will energize you, and it will encourage mobility and good circulation, maintain a healthy weight gain, and promote good posture. If you have exercised prior to pregnancy, you will have increased your blood volume and developed a strong diaphragm, improving your aerobic capability.

Pregnancy is not the time to start doing aerobic exercise to get fit. If you already do it, you can continue if you don't want to let your fitness level drop, but there are guidelines you should follow. Your heart rate should never be raised above 140 beats a minute, and strenuous exercise shouldn't last longer than 15 minutes at a stretch.

SEX IN PREGNANCY

Some women worry that sexual intercourse poses a risk during pregnancy. I don't recommend that you have sex in the first 12 weeks if you are prone to bleeding in early pregnancy or if you have had IVF. You can, however, be intimate in other ways.

Changing hormones, weight gain, decreased energy levels, and debilitating symptoms such as nausea may diminish your sexual desire in the first trimester, but don't worry, this will pass. Make sure you talk to your partner about how you are feeling.

Aim for 20 to 30 minutes' exercise three or four times a week. And remember to relax for the same amount of time as you have exercised.

Benefits for your baby

Exercise causes an increase in your blood volume. This encourages your baby's growth as you boost blood circulation to the baby, promoting the development of fetal tissue. Doing exercise also causes the environment in the uterus to change, providing the baby with a physical challenge to which it can practice its response. In addition, when a mother exercises, not only does her heart rate change but so do her blood-sugar and oxygen levels. This changes the baby's blood, too, and will help it adapt to the rigors of birth, as well as developing its sensitivity to motion, vibration, and different sounds.

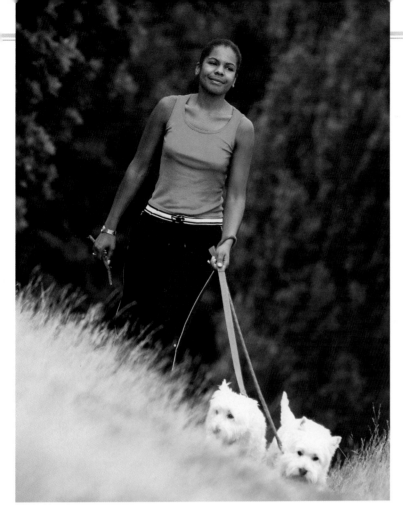

"walking is an excellent form of exercise during pregnancy"

What's good, what's not

Most pregnancy exercise classes are carefully structured, so take care if you go to an ordinary class. Ideally, any exercise should be supervised by a teacher who understands the physiological changes in pregnancy (*see* page 81). Avoid contact sports such as hockey or lacrosse because of the speed and risk of injury. Gentle cycling is good; walking is excellent; and speed walking is preferable to running. Swimming and water-based exercise are good in the second and third trimesters.

If you experience bleeding, breathlessness, dizziness, faintness, or any pain, stop exercising immediately and consult your doctor. You should discuss exercise with your doctor if you are anemic, have had a previous miscarriage, or suffer joint or back problems. I don't recommend any exercise during the first trimester if you've had IVF.

DEALING WITH STRESS

We have already discussed the many concerns in early pregnancy that can cause anxiety. A certain amount of the stress hormone cortisol is needed by the baby for maturing organs such as the lungs, kidneys, liver, and the immune system. However, elevated levels may slow its growth, trigger premature birth, and even give it a heightened cortisol response to stress all its life.

How you deal with stress will make a difference to the health of your unborn child. It is able to detect how stressed you are by the amount of stress hormones that cross the placenta. Its development will alter so that it can react to it. Make a commitment to set aside time every day for a stress-relieving activity. The right breathing technique (*see* page 25) is a start, and if you want to focus your mind more, use visualization (*see* page 67).

prenatal tests

Many women today wait until they get the result of their first prenatal test before sharing the news that they are pregnant. Screening tests determine the level of risk of an abnormality being present, while diagnostic tests, which are invasive and used less commonly, confirm whether there is a problem or not.

ROUTINE CHECKS

Your first prenatal appointment may be as early as 6 or 8 weeks. Your health, medical, and gynecological history will be noted and your dates calculated. A blood sample will be analyzed to determine your blood group and rhesus (Rh) type (*see* page 99); to assess hemoglobin levels for anemia; to screen for infections, such as hepatitis B, syphilis or HIV; and to establish immunity to rubella.

After your first prenatal visit, each time you go for a checkup you will be weighed, your blood pressure will be checked, and your urine will be tested for infection, glucose, and protein. At 28 weeks, your blood will be tested again for anemia and screened for infections, and you will be given a glucose tolerance test.

Dating ultrasound scan

At 11–13 weeks a dating scan may be offered if you haven't had one earlier. This will identify if twins are present, and will use fetal measurements to confirm the exact stage of the pregnancy. The fetal heartbeat will also be checked.

SCREENING TESTS

Noninvasive screening tests gauge the risk of many types of abnormality being present.

Types of screening

• **Nuchal translucency scan**
During an ultrasound scan (*see* pages 74–5) carried out at 11–13 weeks, the fluid under the skin at the back of the baby's neck— the nuchal translucency—is measured. The greater the depth of fluid, the higher the risk of Down syndrome.

• **Combined test** At about 11–13 weeks, the result of a blood test is combined with a nuchal scan measurement to estimate the chances of a baby having Down syndrome.

• **Serum tests** Various tests are used to measure two, three, or more substances in your blood to help predict whether your baby is at risk of Down syndrome, certain other genetic abnormalities, or a neural tube defect (NTD), such as spina bifida.

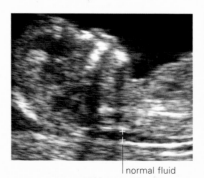
normal fluid

Less than 3mm of fluid behind the neck indicates a low risk of Down syndrome.

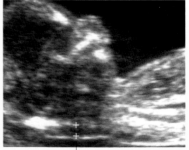
increased fluid

A depth of 4–7mm of fluid puts the fetus at a higher risk of Down syndrome.

Understanding the results

If the result of your screening test is "screen negative," it means the chance of your having a baby with Down syndrome is less than 1 in 250. But that does not rule it out. If the result is "screen positive," the chance is greater than 1 in 250, so you will be offered a diagnostic test. It is your choice whether or not to have one (*see* below).

It is very hard for couples today because there are more tests and more decisions to make at every stage of pregnancy. As a result, some women's anxiety levels go through the roof as they constantly look to scans for reassurance. Try not to focus too much on having tests and getting the results. Trust in your body's natural ability to carry and nurture a healthy baby.

DIAGNOSTIC TESTS

Diagnostic tests are not routine since they are invasive and can cause complications. They will, however, tell you categorically whether or not your baby has an abnormality. Discuss the tests with your midwife or doctor so that you are fully aware of the risks, if any, and the implications.
• **Chorionic villus sampling** (CVS) can be done from 11 weeks onward, and involves the extraction of a sample of tissue from the placenta using the same technique as amniocentesis (*see* box). CVS tests only for chromosomal disorders so serum

AMNIOCENTESIS

Amniocentesis involves passing a needle through the mother's abdomen and removing a sample of amniotic fluid (10–20ml). An ultrasound probe is used to ensure that the needle doesn't touch the fetus or the placenta. Although local anesthetic is placed on the mother's skin, she may feel slight discomfort during the procedure and be a little bit sore afterward.

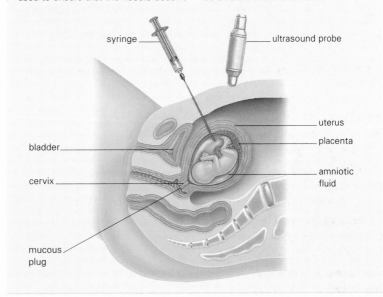

screening for NTDs may be required. The test has a 1 percent risk of miscarriage.
• **Amniocentesis** is usually done at about 16 weeks. A sample of amniotic fluid is removed (*see* box) and analyzed for chromosomal disorders and NTDs (results take up to four weeks). It carries less than 1 percent risk of miscarriage.
• **Cordocentesis** is also known as fetal blood sampling. A sample of the baby's blood is taken from the umbilical cord after 18 weeks, under ultrasound guidance. This is the quickest method of detecting chromosomal abnormalities. It is also used to test for rubella or toxoplasmosis infection in later pregnancy. The risk of miscarriage is 1–2 percent, so the test is undertaken only in specialist units.

DEALING WITH BAD NEWS

It comes as a huge blow when a problem is detected. Knowing that your pregnancy may not continue or that your baby will have a disability is very difficult. There is a lot of information available, as well as counseling or support groups to help you cope with the consequences of whatever you decide to do.

connect with your baby

Your baby does not really start to grow until it has communicated with you. A few days after implantation, the preplacenta cells send chemical "messages" to your ovaries and pituitary gland to announce that you are pregnant. So, right from the start, your baby takes an active role.

THE POWER OF POSITIVE THOUGHT

Many women I see are frightened of connecting with their babies in the early stages of pregnancy, especially if they have undergone an assisted fertility procedure such as IVF. They feel that they might be tempting fate if they dare to believe the baby is really there. But I encourage them to use visualization (*see* opposite) to encourage positive thinking even before the fertilized embryo has been put back in the uterus, and I urge them to continue doing so throughout early pregnancy. I want those of you reading this book to do the same. Don't spend the first few weeks looking for signs that things are not going well and worrying about what might go wrong.

No matter what your gynecological history is or your age, I want you to abandon negative thinking and rid yourself of thoughts such as "I dare not hope that everything will be OK" or "I'm not going to think about the baby until after I've had the test results and I know everything is fine". I understand why women think this way. Not connecting makes them think that, if for any reason they do lose the pregnancy, it will be less

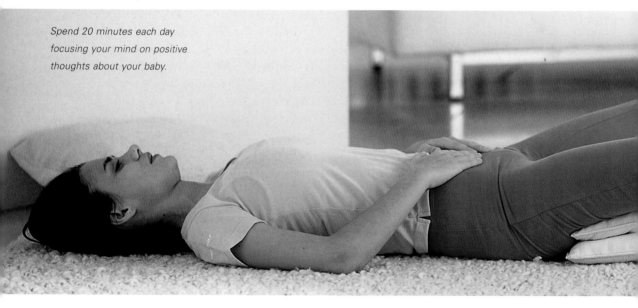

Spend 20 minutes each day focusing your mind on positive thoughts about your baby.

traumatic. But believe me, the disappointment will be just as great. It's important to start connecting now: your baby is!

Any emotion can nourish or deplete your nervous system. Negative thoughts or anxiety provoke a response in your body and trigger the release of stress hormones; joyful thoughts encourage the production of endorphins; while peaceful thoughts have a tranquilizing effect. Your body and therefore your baby are a reflection of your experiences. Remember, throughout your pregnancy, as your baby develops, it is aware of your sensations. If you are happy, sad, anxious, or calm, it is detected in the uterine environment and picked up by your baby's nervous system. Being aware of this and connecting with your baby from the beginning of your pregnancy is the key to creating a nurturing environment conducive to healthy growth.

MAKING TIME FOR THE TWO OF YOU

Call me old-fashioned but, having been a midwife for 25 years, I remember when all pregnant women used to put their feet up in the afternoon and have a rest. A quiet time set aside for deep

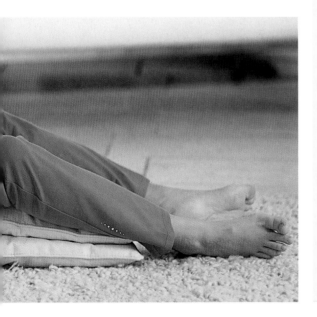

breathing, relaxation, and visualization is so important because you are lying still; blood is not rushing to your extremities so more can be directed to the placenta and uterus.

Talking to your baby sounds slightly eccentric I know, but soon your baby will be able to hear quite well and will respond to music and the sound of familiar voices. Verbalizing your plans and hopes to your baby will familiarize it with your voice. Spending time together and focusing on the baby is very important. Understanding what your baby senses, feels, and experiences and the rhythms of its existence in the uterus (*see* pages 84–5) will help you do this.

FOCUS ON VISUALIZATION

Visualization is a powerful tool used by many athletes to enhance their performance. It can be used in conjunction with hypnotherapy to improve mind-set. I see many women stuck in a negative mind-set in early pregnancy. They are anxious about having scans or, if they've had a miscarriage previously, they doubt their ability to carry a baby to term.

● Lie on your back with your hands resting gently on your abdomen and focus your mind on your uterus.

● Imagine your baby's heart beating strongly. Visualize the placenta as a root system, transporting vital nutrients and oxygen to sustain your baby and establish the foundations of its growth.

● Let go of any other thoughts that enter your mind. Convey thoughts of how much you want this baby.

● This form of exercise is like meditation: it will help calm and relax you. It is a way of staying focused and clearing out unwanted thoughts. Do this connection exercise for 20 minutes a day during the first trimester, either in the morning or in the evening.

● There is no set formula for connecting with your baby; we each have our own level of receptiveness. Some of you will close your eyes and easily be able to conjure up images. If you find it difficult, look at a scan picture or an image in this book depicting the stage you are at in your pregnancy.

expecting more than one

More women are having twins—or more—than a couple of decades ago. Many multiple births result from fertility treatments. You may also have an increased chance of conceiving twins if you're older; if twins run in your family; and if you've had previous pregnancies.

GETTING USED TO THE IDEA

No one is sure why identical twins occur, but a dominant maternal gene may cause a single fertilized egg to split. Fraternal (dizygotic) twins are easier to explain because they tend to run in families or occur when fertility treatment boosts the number of eggs released or when two or more fertilized eggs are returned to the uterus during IVF (*see* page 45).

The news that you're expecting twins (or more) can come as a huge shock, but you'll soon move on to practical considerations such as how you will manage, especially if you already have children; whether or not you'll be able to work; and how will your pregnancy be affected by the fact that you're carrying more than one baby.

There is no doubt that multiple pregnancies can be more difficult, and put you into the category of a "high risk" pregnancy. In the first trimester, you'll be more tired; you'll get bigger quicker; and what may just be minor ailments with a singleton, such as morning sickness, will be exacerbated with twins. But with good nutrition and thorough prenatal care, your babies will thrive.

DIAGNOSING TWINS

Many women, especially those who have had IVF, feel sicker earlier and are incredibly tired if they are expecting more than one baby. You may have elevated levels of human chorionic gonadotropin (HCG)—the hormone detectable in a pregnant

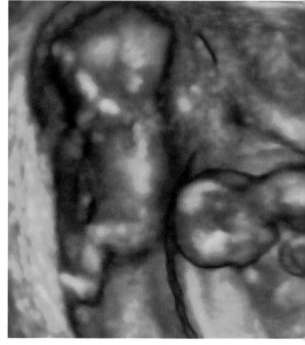

Two babies are clearly visible on this ultrasound image, confirming the presence of a multiple pregnancy.

woman's blood or urine about 10 days after conception. An ultrasound scan will confirm that you are expecting twins or more. If two hearts are detected, or two sacs or placentas are visible, then it's twins! If it can also be seen that they are of a different sex, then you will know they're fraternal rather than identical (monozygotic).

LIFESTYLE ADJUSTMENTS

It is even more important that you rest as much as possible right from the start. You may well have to reduce your work load, cut out traveling—at least at peak times—and you will almost certainly have to start your maternity leave earlier.

There is no reason for you not to exercise as long as you observe the usual precautions: don't get overheated and don't take up anything new or too energetic.

NUTRITION AND WEIGHT GAIN

In a twin pregnancy, how well you eat is the one thing that is under your control, and it has become clear from recent research into reducing preterm labor that maternal nutrition and optimal weight gain are crucial to a good outcome. Poor nutrition is increasingly linked to obstetric complications and, as one medical journal has put it, "multiple gestation is a major nutritional stress."

Women of normal weight who are expecting twins are usually advised to gain 35–45lb (16–20kg) compared with 25–35lb (11–16kg) for a single baby. Women pregnant with triplets should probably expect to gain 50–60lb (23–27kg). A gain of at least 24lb (11kg) by the 24th week of a twin pregnancy will help reduce the risk of having preterm and low-birthweight babies. Early weight gain is particularly important because it will encourage the development of the placenta(s), improving nutrition for babies whose gestation is likely to be shorter.

In the US, women with multiple pregnancies are advised to consume about 300 more calories a day than women carrying one baby—2,700–2,800 calories a day in total. But discuss your specific requirements with your doctor or midwife. Without sufficient calories, you won't have enough energy for the activities of day-to-day life, let alone for building babies.

Adequate protein is needed for building extra body tissue and for keeping your babies' bodies growing and functioning properly. It also plays an important role in creating enough blood volume for you. The recommended amount of protein for a twin pregnancy is at least 4oz (110g) a day; for triplets, it's 5oz (150g)—*see* page 134 for good food sources of protein. By the end of a twin pregnancy your blood volume will have increased by 50 percent, and even more in a triplet pregnancy. This will be achieved partly by increasing your level of hydration (drinking enough fluids) and partly due to adequate protein intakes. Good blood-volume expansion is vitally important for the nourishment of your babies.

It is essential to take a prenatal vitamin and mineral supplement if you discover you are carrying twins or more, and this should contain at least 30mg of iron. More iron is needed for making hemoglobin for the increased numbers of blood cells carrying oxygen—*see* page 135 for good food sources. Iron-deficiency anemia is common in multiple pregnancies: it causes extreme fatigue in the mother and decreased oxygen supply to the babies, and may increase the risk of preterm delivery. If you are diagnosed as anemic you will probably be prescribed an iron supplement.

MONITORING MULTIPLES

You will be monitored more when you are expecting twins than you would be during a single pregnancy. You'll have regular blood tests to check iron and glucose levels and, later in the pregnancy, for signs of more serious complications (*see* pages 106–7), and you'll have scans to monitor the positions of the babies and the placenta(s). Women expecting more than one baby are at an increased risk of gestational hypertension, gestational diabetes, intrauterine growth restriction, an incompetent cervix, and preeclampsia. Close monitoring will allow early detection and management of any problems. Prenatal surveillance such as nonstress fetal heart rate testing (NST; *see* page 107) usually starts between 32 and 34 weeks in twins that are not growing normally, but earlier if other tests give cause for concern.

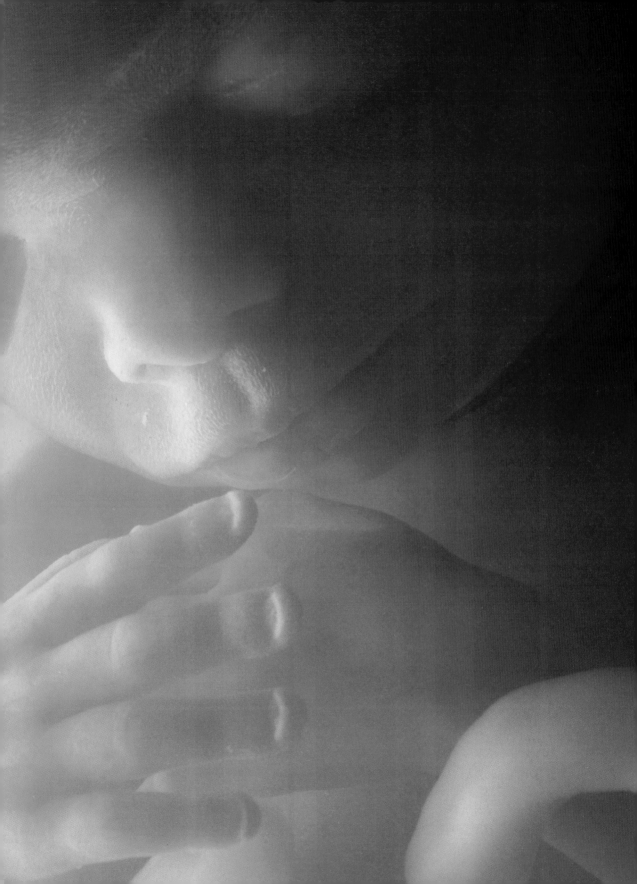

SECOND TRIMESTER
what's happening?

All your baby's organs have developed and in this trimester they will continue to grow. The placenta is getting bigger and thicker. Cushioned by amniotic fluid, your baby is fully active —soon you will start to feel flutters of movement.

FETAL MOVEMENTS

Your baby began to move in the first trimester, as early as 7–8 weeks. This movement is important throughout pregnancy to exercise muscles and prevent joints from seizing up. It is also important in the development of the nervous system, making connections with the brain and spinal cord, and for strengthening and shaping bones.

At first, the baby's movements were smooth and wormlike; by eight weeks there were rapid, irregular movements of the whole body with bending and extending of the trunk and limbs. By nine weeks, the whole body was able to curl up. Isolated arm movements and leg movements began at 9½ weeks and the head started to turn from side to side at 10 weeks, when thumb-sucking also started. Jaw opening and stretching movements started at about 11 weeks; yawning and swallowing at about 13 weeks.

By 15 weeks, stimuli on your abdomen will produce a startle response. At 16 weeks there is good limb coordination and the hands may be clasped. From now on you may be able to feel your baby move—this is known as quickening.

In addition to limb movements, the baby practices breathing. There is no air to breathe, but the fetus breathes in the fluid surrounding it.

By 22 weeks your baby's face and hands are clearly defined. It will practice breathing movements and you may feel it hiccup.

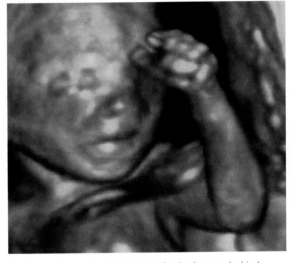

By 17 weeks your baby is very active in the womb. Limb coordination is good and it can open and close its hands.

Breathing movements started as early as 10 weeks and don't stop until life ends. This practice is important to develop the diaphragm and the abdomen and rib muscles, all used in breathing. Lung tissue also needs movement in order to mature. By 22 weeks your baby may hiccup.

GROWTH AND DEVELOPMENT

At 13 weeks, the fetus is about 3in (8cm) in length and weighs about 1oz (25g). By the 17th week, it will have grown to about 5in (13cm) and will weigh about 5oz (150g).

Glucose is satisfying most of your baby's energy needs and at least as much again is being used by the placenta, which is why "good baby carbs" are so important (*see* page 60). Your baby's metabolic processes generate heat that raises the temperature in utero. Its heartbeat is twice as fast as your own.

Weeks 13–16

Your baby's growth is rapid now. Its head is proportionately smaller in relation to the body than it was at 12 weeks. The bones are clearly visible. The limbs are fully formed and the joints can move. The ovaries in female babies contain follicles. Your baby is starting to lay down fat.

Weeks 17–20

"Brown" fat forms from 17 weeks: this burns calories for energy, produces heat, and insulates the baby. The baby is getting heavier and lengthening. The ovaries in a female baby or testes in a male baby are now fully formed. By 20 weeks there is a covering of fine downy hair, and thicker hair is appearing on the head. Fingerprints are starting to form as ridges. The hands can grip firmly and teeth buds are developing.

Weeks 21–25

Substantial weight gain continues. Rapid eye movements begin, and taste has also developed by this stage. From 24 weeks the baby may show definite responses—mainly by variations in heart rate. For example, at about 25 weeks the fetus can open and close its eyes, and responds to a bright light shone on the abdomen with a change in its heart rate and by turning away.

By now all the parts of the ear are complete and, provided the nerve connections are in place, your baby can hear. It used to be thought that external sounds were muffled by the amniotic fluid or obscured by the gurglings of the mother's body. But it is now known that external voices close up, particularly raised voices, can be heard, and the mother's voice is a prominent sound in the uterus.

By 28 weeks

There are now fat deposits beneath the baby's skin, which is covered with a waxy substance called vernix to protect it from its damp surroundings. The lungs are continuing to develop. There is less room for your baby to move and you will be very aware of its activity.

THE AMNIOTIC FLUID

Human beings spend their first nine months in water, harking back to their evolutionary ancestors' aquatic existence. The fluid surrounding a baby in the amniotic sac acts as a cushion in case of impact, protects the baby from infection, allows it to move around, and helps the development of the respiratory, digestive, and musculoskeletal systems.

The liquid is full of suspended flakes. Some of these are waste products from the baby's gut; others are clumps of cells expelled from the baby's lungs. There are also flakes of skin cells floating in the liquid. The cells in the fluid are used to determine the chromosomal status of your baby if you decide or are advised to have an amniocentesis.

In early pregnancy, the amount of fluid in the sac is small, but it increases every day, allowing greater freedom of movement for the fetus. In the first trimester the baby absorbs fluid through its skin, but, after the development of the kidneys in the second trimester, fluid is swallowed, passed through the gut and kidneys, and excreted as perfectly sterile urine before being consumed again. Fluid is also taken into the lungs, and the right amount of fluid is important for their development. At the start of the second trimester there is probably about a cupful (200ml) of fluid.

The amniotic fluid is vitally important for your baby's development. If the amniotic sac ruptures in early pregnancy and the fluid is lost, it is rare for the baby to survive.

HOW YOUR BODY IS CHANGING

Many women are desperate for their babies to start showing. By the end of 12 weeks, your uterus is starting to rise above the pubic bone; by 16 weeks, it is between the pubic bone and the belly button; by 24 weeks it is at your belly button. These measurements help your midwife and doctor to gauge how your baby is developing and growing. Skin pigmentation is common: the areola around your nipples may be the first to change, becoming darker. Many women develop a linea nigra, or black line, extending down the center of the abdomen. From the point of view of physical symptoms, most women start to feel much better in the second trimester.

BRAIN DEVELOPMENT

Although the nervous system is still relatively immature, its foundations are in place by about 16–18 weeks. The earliest recorded brain activity is at seven weeks, corresponding to the first fetal movements. Brainwaves become more regular about 10 weeks. The first distinguishing of brainwave type (which depends on wavelength) occurs at 20 weeks.

Your baby's brain cells (neurons) are multiplying at a rate of 250,000 a minute. These cells are connected by millions of axons—the long extensions from neurons that transmit nerve impulses from the cell bodies—like wiring from circuits. By week 25 most of the axons have arrived at their destinations so the basic neural network is in place.

During development the brain produces twice as many cells and the baby needs. Billions of cells are loosely wired and need to be stimulated to make connections with other cells. The excess that are not stimulated won't connect and will die. This is a natural process that happens at around eight months, so don't wait until your baby is born to start maximizing its potential brain power—the more connections there are, the fewer the number of brain cells that will die.

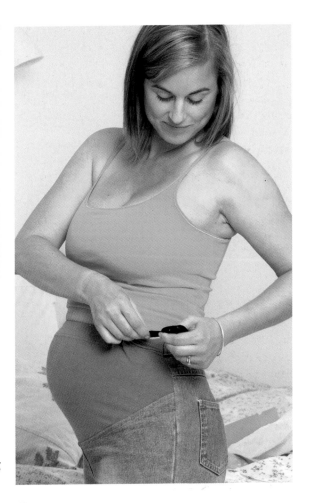

"many women are desperate for their babies to start showing"

ultrasound scans

Ultrasound scanning is routinely used to monitor the growth and development of your baby during pregnancy. It is also used to identify "markers" that indicate possible chromosomal abnormalities. Between 18 and 21 weeks, detailed scanning can pick up major malformations as well as some minor ones.

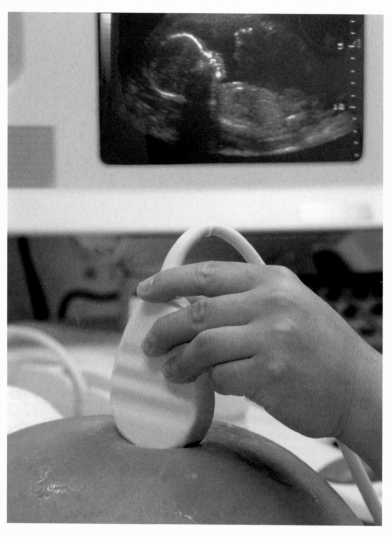

A QUESTION OF TIMING

Early scans (up to 10 weeks) are recommended if a problem is suspected; if there is a history of early pregnancy failure; if dates are uncertain; or for women who have had assisted fertility procedures (the risk of ectopic pregnancy increases with IVF).

First trimester scans (10–14 weeks) are usually offered to assess size for dates and as part of the screening for Down syndrome (*see* page 64) and fetal abnormalities.

A second trimester scan (18–21 weeks) is commonly done to check the development of the baby. In particular, the heart, kidneys, brain, and spine and limbs will be checked, and the growth of the head, body, and limbs will be measured. The position of the placenta will also be noted.

Third trimester scans (32–36 weeks) assess the baby's size and weight, its position, and the condition and position of the placenta prior to delivery.

FETAL MEASUREMENTS

The circumferences of the head and abdomen and the length of the femur (thigh bone) are measured and the relationship between them gives a key indication of growth.

Head circumference

By the end of the first trimester, the baby's head is 30 percent of the size it will be at term. By 20 weeks it's about half its final size, and by 28 weeks three-quarters. The growth of the head corresponds to the growth of the brain, which takes precedence over other parts of the body. So if the baby's overall growth is adversely affected during the second half of pregnancy, the head grows at the expense of the abdomen and femur (*see* page 78).

Abdominal circumference

This measurement is closely related to fetal weight: the abdomen grows faster during the second half of pregnancy than it does during the first. Abdominal circumference includes fat and carbohydrate stores in the liver, both of which decline if growth is restricted.

By the end of 12 weeks the baby's weight is only 3 percent of what it will be at term; by 20 weeks it's 9 percent, but by 28 weeks it's nearly 75 percent.

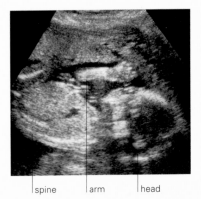

spine   arm   head

A routine scan at about 20 weeks; measurements will help assess growth.

Femur length

The length of the thigh bone provides a good barometer of long-term growth. Growth is faster during the second half of pregnancy than the first.

FREQUENTLY ASKED QUESTIONS

How does ultrasound scanning work?
A small, handheld ultrasound probe (transducer) is passed over the abdomen, beaming high-frequency sound waves into the body tissues. Echoes produced as the pulses strike structures are converted into electrical signals, which are processed to produce an image.

Is ultrasound safe?
There is no evidence that scanning harms either mother or baby, but there are strict guidelines for its use during pregnancy, purely as a precaution.

Do I really need to have scans?
Ultrasound scanning plays an important role in many pregnancies. It confirms viability in the first few months; it can detect most fetal abnormalities; it identifies disorders that might put the baby at risk; it assesses a baby's welfare during late pregnancy and helps determine the timing of delivery in high-risk pregnancies.

Does ultrasound scanning detect all fetal abnormalities?
Even expert ultrasonographers can miss an abnormality, and certain anomalies cannot be picked up by scan. However, the detection rate for anencephaly (brain defect), for example, is 98 percent and for spina bifida is 80 percent.

Can ultrasound detect Down syndrome babies?
Ultrasound scanning screens for all types of chromosomal disorders, in particular Down syndrome. The scan measures the thickness of skin at the back of the baby's neck—the nuchal thickness (*see* page 64). Combined with a blood test, the scan gives a detection rate of 80–90 percent, but a diagnostic test is then needed to confirm Down syndrome.

What is transvaginal scanning?
A narrow ultrasound probe is inserted into the vagina. This provides higher-quality imaging of the uterus and pelvis, allowing first trimester confirmation of normal development; more accurate heart monitoring; and improved detection of pregnancy complications, such as an ectopic pregnancy.

good eating plan

There are various important nutrients that are in great demand at this stage of pregnancy because they are involved in building your baby's skeleton. Insufficient intakes may result in abnormal development of bones and teeth.

CALCIUM

Calcium is needed throughout pregnancy, but it is especially important in the second trimester for your baby's bones (*see* pages 76–7). If your intake is low, calcium from your own bones will be used to meet your baby's needs, a process that can weaken them. Calcium also helps keep blood pressure normal and may reduce the risk of preterm delivery. Pay carefull attention to your calcium intake during this trimester. For optimum absorption of calcium from food or supplements, you need adequate supplies of vitamins C and D and phosphorus.

PHOSPHORUS

Phosphorus is second only to calcium as the most abundant mineral in the body. It is essential for the overall development of your baby and to support the pregnancy; it's necessary for cell growth and for healthy muscles and bones. It is part of all cells so it is available in all major food groups.

VITAMIN D

Vitamin D, or calciferol, is a fat-soluble vitamin. It is found in food, but also can be made in the body after exposure to the sun's ultraviolet rays. The major biological function of vitamin D is to maintain normal blood levels of calcium and phosphorus. I encourage 20 minutes of sunlight a day to help build up your body's reserves of vitamin D. Go out in the sun safely: for a few minutes at a time, or at the beginning or end of the day in midsummer when the sun is strong.

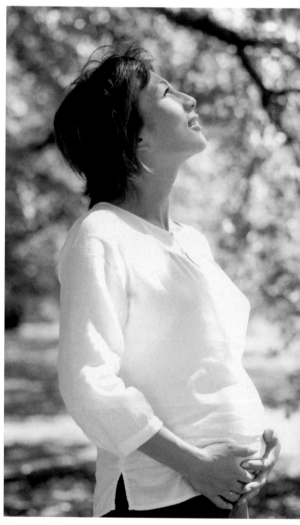

The ultraviolet rays in sunlight trigger vitamin D synthesis in the skin—make sure you get 20 minutes of sunlight a day.

ZINC

Zinc is required for protein and essential fatty acid metabolism and cell development. Think zinc for optimum growth. It is involved in a hundred different enzyme reactions, many of which are concerned with growth. Low levels usually mean smaller babies and may be linked to learning difficulties.

MAGNESIUM

Seventy percent of the magnesium in the body is found in bones and teeth. It is the third most common mineral in body cells and it is important for every major metabolic reaction, as well as for helping regulate the heart.

IRON

Being low in iron will make you tired, more prone to infections, and may result in a more difficult labor and birth. Ultimately, you could also suffer from anemia. The body conserves iron during pregnancy, but stores still dwindle because the fetus draws on your iron supplies to create its own supply.

Iron is necessary for hemoglobin, the substance in red blood cells that enables transportation of oxygen. It also helps the immune system function properly and is critical for normal brain function. Eating at least three servings of iron-rich foods a day should ensure that you get enough iron in your daily diet (*see* page 135). If possible, iron should not be taken with calcium or magnesium, either

WEIGHT WATCH

You need to eat an extra 300 calories a day in the second trimester because your baby is growing rapidly. This equates to a sandwich or a bowl of cereal, so it's not a great deal. Gaining about 1lb (450g) a week is a good sign that you're getting enough calories. Many women are surprised at how hungry they are during the second trimester, but the placenta is producing hormones that will stimulate your appetite so that you eat enough to fuel the baby's growth.

of which may decrease absorption. Caffeine also inhibits iron absorption. It is better absorbed when taken with foods high in vitamin C. Iron is lost in cooking, so cook vegetables in a small amount of water and for the shortest possible time.

ESSENTIAL FATTY ACIDS

Your baby cannot make its own essential fatty acids (EFAs), such as DHA (*see* page 21), and is dependent on you for its supply. Unless you are eating 1oz (30g) of nuts and seeds a day and 10oz (300g) of oily fish a week, neither you nor your baby is likely to be getting enough. EFAs are particularly important for brain development. At around 24 weeks the baby's eyes are developing and light-sensitive cells in the retina start to accumulate more and more EFAs.

In a subsequent pregnancy women are advised to take DHA supplements because their DHA levels tend to be lower than in first pregnancies.

FOOD ALLERGIES

More and more people are becoming sensitive to common foods that are important sources of nutrients during pregnancy—dairy products, wheat, eggs, and nuts, for example. There is now good evidence that sensitization may occur in utero, possibly as early as 22 weeks. Allergens may cross the placenta from the mother and one theory is that the fetus may respond to these because, due to better hygiene, there are fewer parasites, for example, for it to respond to.

Boosting your immune system will help. If allergies run in your family or that of your partner, avoid eating foods that are commonly implicated while you're pregnant. Alternatively, rotate common allergens such as dairy products with, for example, goat's milk products so that your baby is not exposed to any one of them too often. This might at least lessen the severity of the baby's reaction.

windows of opportunity
growth and bones

Your baby has several growth spurts during the second trimester. Poor nutrition from the third to the sixth months of pregnancy will result in the baby being thinner and having a reduced birthweight, smaller head circumference, poor brain development, and an increased risk of certain diseases in later life.

VARIATIONS IN GROWTH RATE

If growth slows in early pregnancy due to infection or low maternal weight, the baby adapts by slowing its overall growth. All measurements begin to reflect below-average growth patterns as the pregnancy develops—and this may be linked to premature labor.

Sometimes fetal growth proceeds normally during the first trimester, but slows during the second if the mother overexerts herself physically, works too hard, gains too little weight, becomes anemic, or gets an infection. The baby is dependent on the placenta for food, water, and oxygen. If it doesn't get the required amounts, it has to adapt by redirecting blood to vital organs.

The baby's weight at birth is then likely to be reduced. This baby will be short or stunted for its gestational age. In infancy its growth will continue to lag behind.

If, for similar reasons, growth slows in the third trimester, the baby adapts by sustaining brain growth at the expense of the rest of the body. Body length and head circumference are normal, but the baby is born very thin.

FOCUS ON BONES

The second trimester is a crucial time for the development of your baby's bones. Bone is a type of connective tissue that is strong but very light. It consists of specialized cells and fibers of protein

CONSEQUENCES OF LOW BIRTH WEIGHT

A baby who is born with good birth weight will generally expend less energy on growth when he or she is a year old, and his or her growth rate will slow down. However, children who were smaller at birth need to catch up, and they will therefore put on weight rapidly. This is known as compensatory growth.

Professor Barker at Southampton University, England, has done a lot of research into the effects of compensatory growth, revealing that nutritionally the effects are not necessarily beneficial. If growth is too fast, nutrients will not be absorbed properly, which will affect body tissues, increasing the workloads of the kidneys

and the pancreas. This in turn may lead to higher blood pressure and possible diabetes in later life. It is also thought that the "deferred costs" of low birth weight followed by catch-up growth in childhood may lead to increased risk of illnesses such as heart disease in later life. Poor diet and lifestyle will compound these effects further.

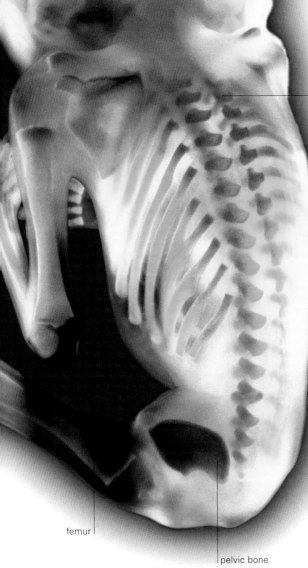

vertebrae

femur

pelvic bone

During the second trimester, fetal bones calcify, drawing hugely on maternal reserves of calcium.

bone cells, known as osteoblasts, make a sort of scaffolding on which calcium salt crystals are deposited, a process known as "mineralization." A baby's bones do not harden fully until after birth and the joints between the skull bones until even later. Bones do not ossify completely until early in adult life when bone growth comes to an end.

Mineralization hardens bone, and if the process doesn't happen at the correct rate, the bones may be weakened. It may not happen properly if a child grows rapidly in infancy or early childhood to compensate for a previous period of slow growth. There is some evidence that improper mineralization in the early years affects the mineral loss that we all experience as we get older, resulting in weak bones that fracture easily, although much research still needs to be done on why osteoporosis develops in later life.

The skeleton of a newborn baby is made up of more than 300 parts. As the baby grows, some of its bones fuse together, and by adulthood the skeleton contains just 206 bones.

As fetal bones begin to calcify (harden) initially, the baby draws on the mineral stores in its mother's bones, and there is a dramatic shift of calcium across the placenta. Adequate calcium is essential for maintaining healthy bones and teeth in a pregnant woman, as well as providing for the skeletal development of the fetus.

Your body adapts to the demands of the fetus and makes calcium available either from your own reserves or by absorbing more during digestion. Make sure that you eat a varied and balanced diet to ensure an adequate intake of this important mineral during this trimester (*see* page 135 for food sources of calcium).

that are interwoven in a kind of matrix made up of water, mineral salts, and carbohydrates. Bone tissue is not rigid, and it continually breaks down and rebuilds during the growing process. At the center of mature bone is the bone marrow, some of which is soft tissue that produces blood cells and some of which is mostly fat tissue; bone also has blood vessels running through it.

Most of a baby's bones develop from cartilage. Ossification is the process by which the cartilage is converted into bone as a result of the deposition of mineral salts, mainly calcium. The specialized

looking at lifestyle

As a general rule, once women get past the first 12 weeks of pregnancy, with unpleasant symptoms and the first scan behind them, they start to feel better. This is when you will really start to believe that you're going to have a baby: you can focus on the pregnancy and start to plan ahead.

WORKING THROUGH PREGNANCY

Many women want to work for as long as possible during pregnancy so they can take off more time after the birth. This is fine as long as you are prepared to slow down if there are signs that you are doing too much. You don't want to risk going into labor exhausted and depleted of energy.

You should also take it easy in the first and second trimesters. Rest as much as you can. At this point, in addition to tolerating symptoms, balancing your blood-sugar levels, and coping with fatigue, you have the stress of traveling to and from work.

Taking care at work

Ask your midwife or doctor about what you should or shouldn't do in your particular circumstances. Discuss risk factors such as excessive heat in the

"be prepared to slow down at work if there are signs that you are doing too much"

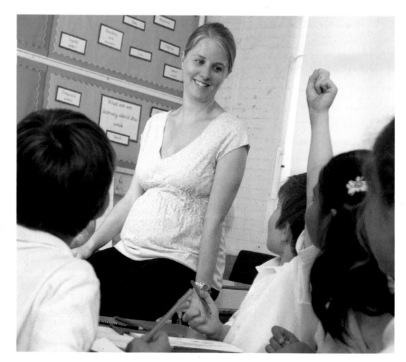

workplace and exposure to hazardous chemicals, radiation, gas or dust, or infectious diseases. While you are at work:
• Change positions often.
• Drink plenty of water and carry high-energy snacks, such as cheese and crackers or a banana.
• Familiarize yourself with the symptoms of late-pregnancy problems (*see* pages 96–9), so that you can read the signs if you're doing too much.

EXERCISE

You need a variety of exercises to work all your muscles and joints. Walking, swimming, and gentle aerobics are good for the circulation and will not put stress on your joints. You may also find you get breathless more easily. Be aware of the physiological changes that occur during pregnancy before you do any exercise.
• The hormone relaxin relaxes ligaments so that the pelvis can expand during delivery. But all other ligaments relax too, so the stability of your joints is affected.
• Due to the effects of progesterone, the diaphragm changes shape and the ribs flare out slightly to allow room for the growing uterus.
• The amount of blood pumped by the heart increases by at least 40 percent during pregnancy and your heart increases in size to cope.
• Increases in girth and weight cause your center of gravity to shift, so you may find it harder to coordinate and balance.
• As body mass increases, it creates momentum, which makes it more difficult to control the direction and pace of movement.

Pilates is good exercise for pregnant women because it consists of controlled movements allowing you time to adjust your posture and alignment. It improves muscular endurance—which is useful during labor and delivery—and strengthens the core abdominal and back muscles, improving your posture, flexibility, and balance.

Yoga also has great benefits during pregnancy. It will increase your sense of well-being, making you

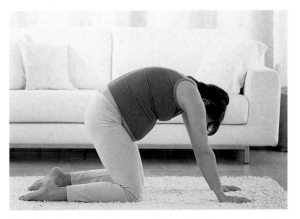

Gentle back-strengthening exercises will help you cope with the ever-increasing load you are carrying in front of you.

more centered and less stressed. With its emphasis on breathing technique and body awareness, it encourages flexibility, boosts circulation, relieves aches and pains, and improves muscle tone in readiness for labor and beyond.

As your weight load increases at the front, you need to take care of your back. Do gentle back-strengthening exercises and think about your posture. Stand up straight, with shoulders back and bottom tucked in, to avoid back strain.

SEX IN THE SECOND TRIMESTER

During the second trimester, you may find your interest in sex changes. Increased blood flow to your sexual organs and breasts may rekindle desire that was depressed during the first few weeks.

MEDITATION

Meditation is an excellent way of using your brainpower more effectively and reducing the inhibiting effects of stress on both mind and body. It is a learned skill for most of us. A course of instruction, or a retreat, might be a good way to learn, but you can try meditation at home, practicing for about 10 or 15 minutes a day. You need to get comfortable and breathe calmly (*see* page 25). Reduce your brain's activity by just letting thoughts come and go.

when learning begins

Until recently, the learning potential of a baby in the uterus was underestimated, especially in the Western world. Eastern philosophies were more sophisticated, giving a newborn the age of one, acknowledging that birth is a milestone in a baby's continuing development.

SENSORY EXPERIENCES

Babies have an instinctive awareness of their surroundings and what they are experiencing while in the uterus. I firmly believe that you can use this awareness to help your baby learn as it develops over the nine months of pregnancy.

While growing in your uterus, your baby is developing its senses and will be capable of seeing, smelling, hearing, feeling, and tasting when born. We talk a lot about stimulating a newborn baby, but in fact this can and should start much sooner. We should be talking to our unborn babies, playing music to them, and finding ways of improving their environment in the uterus.

The brain is the most complex organ and it develops rapidly as the pregnancy progresses. By 20 weeks the neural network is sophisticated. Your baby is starting to kick and communicate with you. It is learning about your world, your habits, your routines, and picking up many stimuli from how you live your life, physically, mentally, and emotionally. In the long term, this will all have an impact on your baby's development.

Hearing

From about the time you feel the first kicks, your baby can hear. The most distinguishable sound is your heartbeat. Your baby is more aware of this than any other sound and it provides a soothing backdrop to everyday life. If you play heartbeat

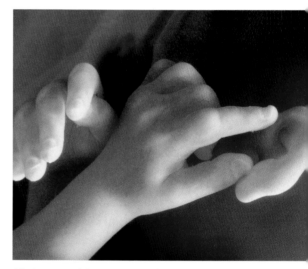

All the parts of the ear needed for hearing are formed by 24 weeks—the most distinguishable sound is your hearbeat.

sounds after the birth, it will calm the baby; cuddling your baby close to your chest has a similar effect. Sounds such as digestive gurglings are loud because they resonate through the amniotic fluid.

Research into the ability of the fetus to hear has provided great insight into the prenatal development of personality and learning (*see* also pages 84–5). All the parts of the ear needed for hearing are formed by 24 weeks, and the baby shows definite responses to sounds, mainly by changes in its heart rate, at between 24 and 26 weeks once the nerve connections are in place. Research suggests that excessive noise during pregnancy may result in high-frequency hearing loss in a newborn, and may be associated with prematurity and intrauterine growth retardation.

Sight

The fetus can open and close its eyes from about 25 weeks. It sees everything inside the uterus in shades of black, gray, and white. (Color vision is not thought to develop until two months after birth.) It responds to bright light shone through the abdomen by turning away and its heart rate increases.

Taste

Tastebuds have developed by six months. Your baby is floating in warm amniotic fluid, which it drinks regularly. The flavor of the fluid varies depending on your diet. Your baby has to get used to various tastes to help it appreciate your milk after birth. Studies show food preferences develop during pregnancy: women who drink a lot of carrot juice have babies who like carrots, for example. This is called dietary imprinting and may have evolved to ensure that babies are born knowing which foods are safe to eat and which are not. Allergies are now thought to be triggered in the uterus (*see* page 77).

Smell

From about 24 weeks, the fetus can also detect the smell of the amniotic fluid. It swallows the fluid and the smell receptors at the top of the nose are bathed in it. Our sense of smell is strongest at birth: a three-day-old baby can instantly recognize the smell of its mother's milk and is greatly soothed by her smell.

Touch

As space in the uterus gets tight, some parts of your baby's body press against the wall of the uterus and it will be aware of gentle pressure.

Throughout pregnancy, and especially during the last three months, your uterus contracts regularly. These tightenings are known as Braxton Hicks contractions. They squeeze the baby and are thought to be an important stimulus for its developing senses and brain as well as helping tone the uterine muscle in preparation for labor. When you stroke or pat your abdomen your baby will sense the stimulus and may quieten down or become alert and respond by kicking.

YOUR BABY'S INTERNAL CLOCK

Your baby is aware of the progression of day and night. Information about the rhythm of the outside world passes from mother to fetus in many ways. Changes in noise level, your eating habits, patterns of exercise, and your relaxation time, all have effects the fetus can monitor. The fetus can also tell what is happening in its mother's world by the amount of cortisol crossing the placenta, and adjusts its own production accordingly. So, if the mother's rhythms are not regular—if she snatches the odd meal here and there, for example—the fetus will receive irregular signals.

Research indicates that a child's sleeping patterns are set in utero by its mother. A Swiss study demonstrated that a group of pregnant early risers bore early-rising babies, while late-nighters produced children that went to bed late. By about 32 weeks, your baby has developed four activity patterns: active sleep, quiet sleep, active awareness, and quiet awareness. Brainwave patterns show that active sleep is similar to rapid eye movement or REM sleep, in which the eyes move constantly and the brain is extremely active. Up to 32 weeks, your baby spends a lot of time in active sleep. After that, it spends more time being aware and awake in the buildup to the birth.

Interestingly, when a premature baby's environment is carefully controlled—in terms of rhythmic components such as lighting, touch, and feeding times—the baby thrives. So, when a baby is in tune with its environment, growth and development are improved. Good lessons in pregnancy— regularity of habit, eating, sleeping, work, and relaxation— will give the baby a better chance of developing normally.

connect with your baby

Sensory experiences and stimulation in the uterus are critical for your baby's normal physical, emotional, and intellectual development. Much of this happens naturally, but there are plenty of things you can do to help.

STIMULATION IN THE UTERUS

Now that your pregnancy is progressing, it is important to start to connect with and stimulate your baby. I believe this can optimize your baby's potential for physical, emotional, and intellectual development. Your baby cannot connect or bond with you on its own: if you shut down emotionally your baby will be adrift. We talk a lot about connecting and bonding after birth, but this should be a continuation of something that started while your baby was still in the uterus. Connect with your baby through touching, talking, singing, and playing music, and you will also be stimulating all of its senses (*see* pages 82–3).

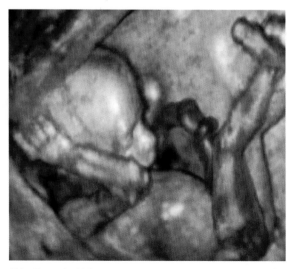

This 17-week-old fetus can be seen wriggling and kicking, probably in response to some form of external stimulus.

Why stimulate your baby?

The aim is to allow your baby to achieve its full potential. You may also boost its intelligence and reduce its risk of being dyslexic or developing attention deficit and hyperactivity disorder (ADHD) along the way. You can help your unborn baby:
• communicate with you and your partner
• differentiate between sounds in the uterus and sounds in the outside world
• learn that sounds have meaning and can be used to communicate; begin the first steps toward developing language through the association of words and meanings
• focus attention; develop and exercise memory
• learn the concept of rhythm.

STARTING TO COMMUNICATE

By interacting with your baby several times a day, you can form a special bond. Babies, both in the uterus and beyond, communicate through movement. Sudden or loud noise will be followed by a kick, showing the baby is distressed. Maternal emotions such as anger, anxiety, and fear may also prompt furious kicking. New studies show that if you experience fear and your heart starts racing, so does your baby's. Conversely, when you read a story to your baby, its heart rate will slow.

Talking to your baby

Your baby hears your voice vibrating through your body. It learns to recognize the tone, speech, and voice patterns that are unique to you, and will

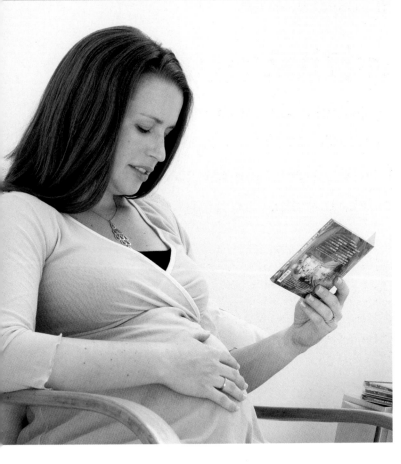

"research shows that prenatal music gives babies a head start"

recognize your voice instantly after birth. The sound of deep male voices passes through the abdominal wall more easily than the sound of female voices. The baby will recognize the male voices heard most frequently but will prefer the sounds of its mother. Combine talking to your baby with rest and relaxation. Set aside 30 minutes or more a day—preferably at the same time—to be in a quiet place alone with your baby and talk.

In addition, you can communicate with your child through touch: whenever you feel a kick, touch the opposite side (where the baby's head is) and caress the area while you speak.

Listening to music

Peter Hepper of Belfast University reported in *The Lancet* the experiences of a group of women who liked to watch the television soap *Neighbours* during pregnancy. They noted that, after their babies were born, if they were irritable, they stopped crying when the programs theme tune came on.

Research also shows that prenatal music gives babies a head start. Yehudi Menuhin had the violin played to him daily when he was in the uterus, and many other musicians describe having had the same "training." Babies whose mothers play classical music to them from 20 weeks onward, for 10 minutes twice a day, seem to develop more quickly and have improved intellectual development.

Singing to soothe

Singing increases lung capacity and relieves stress, both of which are useful preparation for labor. It will improve your sense of well-being, which will be passed on to your baby, and provides a means of prelinguistic communication, helping you bond. The baby will remember the songs after birth and may be soothed by them.

expecting more than one

By now you will look far more advanced in your pregnancy—up to six or eight weeks ahead—than a woman carrying a single baby. Adequate rest is vitally important to help you avoid complications that are more common in multiple pregnancies.

HEALTH COMPLICATIONS

At least 50 percent of twin pregnancies progress normally and result in the birth of two healthy babies. Nevertheless, multiple pregnancies are regarded as "higher risk" because the chance of complications is statistically higher compared with single pregnancies, so you will be monitored more if you are expecting more than one (*see* pages 68–9).

If a problem develops, it will be managed to allow the pregnancy to continue for as long as possible. If it gets worse, it may be necessary to induce labor or to schedule a cesarean section.

High blood pressure

Women expecting multiples are more likely to develop high blood pressure: about 30 percent, compared with 10 percent of women carrying one baby. Pregnancy-induced hypertension is also more common in first pregnancies, women having a subsequent baby but with a new partner, teenage mothers, women over 35 years old, and those with a family history of high blood pressure.

Gestational diabetes

Women with a multiple pregnancy are two to three times more likely (6–9 percent) to develop diabetes, compared with singletons (less than 3 percent). This increased likelihood is thought to be due to higher levels of placental hormones. Diabetes is also more common in women with a family history of the disease, women who are overweight, and women over 35.

Cervical weakness

This can be a problem in any pregnancy, and can result in late miscarriage. In multiple pregnancies the pressure exerted on the cervix is inevitably greater. The 20-week scan will check how the cervix is performing. If it is starting to shorten and dilate, a cervical stitch might be considered to help keep the babies in. You will need to avoid strenuous activity and rest as much as possible during the remainder of the pregnancy. The stitch is removed at about 37 weeks.

Cord entanglement

If identical twins share one amniotic sac, there is a risk of their umbilical cords becoming entangled. This is a potentially life-threatening situation if blood supplies are restricted or even cut off. The cords are monitored at regular intervals by scanning, and the babies are often delivered by cesarean section to avoid cord problems during delivery.

Too much amniotic fluid

A condition more common for identical multiples is excessive amniotic fluid surrounding one or both babies. This may be because there is twin-to-twin transfusion (*see* facing page), or because of a physical or genetic abnormality, but in most cases the cause is unknown. It can develop quite rapidly, typically around the middle of the pregnancy, and may cause miscarriage or very premature birth. An attempt may be made to remove fluid using a technique similar to amniocentesis.

Bleeding during pregnancy

Bleeding beyond 20 weeks of pregnancy may indicate problems with the placenta (*see* pages 96–9), such as placenta previa. With multiple pregnancies, there may be either more than one placenta or a larger amount of placental tissue to support the babies, increasing the chances of the placenta lying lower in the uterus.

Premature birth

A birth is described as "premature" if it is before 37 weeks. About 50 percent of twins are born prematurely; about 80–90 percent of triplets; and virtually all quadruplets (or more). This compares with about 7 percent of single babies. Labor may start spontaneously or you may have to be induced or have an early cesarean section because of complications. If this occurs before 34 weeks, you will need to go to a hospital with a neonatal intensive care unit (NICU).

Reduced birth weight

In general, twins grow at much the same rate as single babies until about 32 weeks. Between 32 to 36 weeks, they gain weight slightly less rapidly, but after 36 weeks' growth can be noticeably less. One twin is usually slightly larger than the other, but if their weight and growth differences are noticeable, there may be concern for the smaller one and the babies may need to be delivered. This may be because blood flow is reduced or because the placenta is providing fewer nutrients.

Twin-to-twin transfusion syndrome (TTTS)

This condition affects only identical twins. It happens when connections form between arteries and veins deep in the placenta, so blood shunts from one baby to another, creating a circulation imbalance. In effect, one twin "donates" its blood to the other. TTTS occurs in up to 17 percent of identical twins sharing a placenta. The physical signs of TTTS can be detected on a scan and are evident before 28 weeks.

BEDREST

The management of several of the conditions that threaten a multiple pregnancy may involve bedrest. This is a matter of degree: full bedrest—just a few trips to the bathroom and most of the time lying on your left side (to improve blood flow to the uterus)—is severely restricting. Modified bedrest may mean that you can sit up for meals or even get out of bed for a few hours a day. Or you may just be confined to the house. Make sure you understand exactly what you can and can't do.

You are bound to find bedrest difficult at times. To keep yourself sane, you need to establish a routine—read the paper; write emails; treat yourself to a new nightgown or a facial; do jobs that you never normally get around to, such as sorting photographs; read, do research, write a journal. Make your bed life as easy as possible—use a table to keep everything within reach, including a means of communicating with everybody else in the house, snacks, and water. Ask others for help, especially if you have other children. Hold on to the fact that it won't last forever.

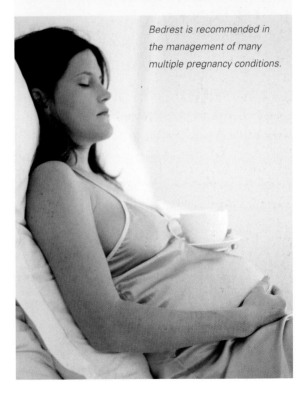

Bedrest is recommended in the management of many multiple pregnancy conditions.

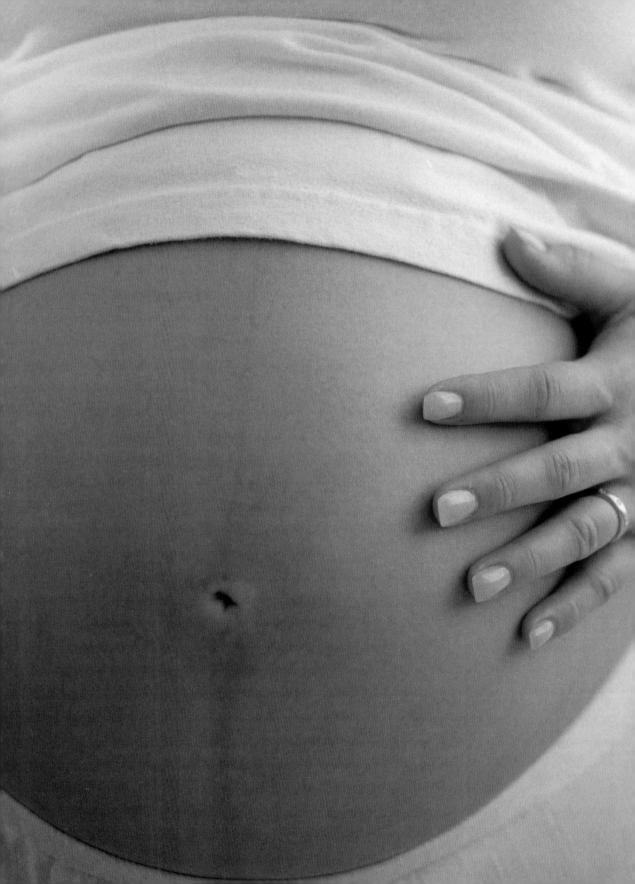

THIRD TRIMESTER
what's happening?

During the third trimester a fetus is undergoing many changes: its growth is dramatic during this period and its organ systems start to mature preparing for the outside world. It also starts to get ready for the challenge of birth.

REHEARSING FOR LIFE

The nervous system continues to become more sophisticated, movements of the muscles more coordinated, and the fetal bone marrow is producing lots of cells. The baby is becoming increasingly aware of its environment.

28–33 weeks

Weight gain is as much as 1lb 2oz (500g) and will continue at a rate of 7–9oz (200–250g) per week between 32 and 35 weeks as your baby lays down fat. On average, babies weigh about 6lb (2.5kg) at 35 weeks.

The mouth and nasal passages are filled with amniotic fluid; the baby processes a pint a day to help the digestive and respiratory systems practice for real-life function. The sucking reflex is also important, ready for breastfeeding. Hiccups are a bit of a mystery, however: one theory is that they help newborns latch onto a nipple.

Taste buds are maturing and your baby will continue to detect flavors from your food when breastfeeding. The eyes will be opening and closing. Bright light may be detectable but the fetus is in darkness. The pigment in your baby's eyes is blue in the uterus, and needs light to change color. This happens in the first weeks

Your bump will grow dramatically during this final trimester. By touching and stroking it you can connect with your baby.

of life if it is going to. The baby hears sound that travels through the fluid four times faster than through air. Its hearing is acute: it can detect sloshing, beats, bumps, and gurglings as well as noises from the world outside.

33 weeks

Your baby may recognize a piece of music by now (*see* pages 84–5) and react to it by kicking. It will have less room for movement now and is asleep up to 90 percent of the time.

35 weeks

Your baby excretes about three-quarters of a quart of urine a day. The amniotic fluid reaches a peak volume of 1¾ pints (1 liter), after which it reduces to as little as 4–7fl oz (100–200ml). Your doctor may monitor fluid levels because they are an indication of growth and kidney problems. Excess fluid is more than 3½ pints (2 liters).

BABY'S MOVEMENTS

You will be aware of strong movements and become attuned to them. Many women worry about how many movements they should be feeling day and night, and your doctor and midwife will ask if you are noting them. It's harder if this is your first baby, of course, because you have nothing to compare it with. And every pregnancy is different in any case. My daughter was much quieter in the uterus and is now serene and calm, whereas my son never stopped moving and still doesn't! Just get used to whatever your baby's pattern of activity is and be mindful of any dramatic change. (Some midwives suggest drinking a glass of cold water if the baby hasn't moved for a while!)

THE PLACENTA

Placental function continues to be of great importance at this stage, and problems with it impact heavily on the pregnancy (*see* pages 96–9). By 30 weeks, the placenta weighs 1lb (450g) and receives 1 pint (500ml) of blood from the mother's circulation every minute. It is limited in the amount of oxygen, glucose, and other nutrients it can deliver to the fetus because it is a major consumer itself of these key fuels (*see* pages 56–7). The placenta has to survive in order for the fetus to survive and has first call on supplies.

The fetus is not connected to its mother by nerves, but there is new evidence that the fetus may be able to influence its environment by the use of hormones produced by the placenta. If it is distressed, hormonal "messages" are sent to the mother, which may indirectly influence her own hormone levels. The separation at birth could conceivably produce a "let down" which may contribute to postpartum depression in susceptible women.

At term, the placenta is flat and round and about 7–8in (18–20cm) in diameter and 1in (2.5cm) thick. It weighs a sixth of the weight of the baby and is divided by grooves into 15 to 20 irregular lobes called cotyledons. Each cotyledon has its own blood supply.

THE LUNGS

By about 29 weeks, most of the small airways, or bronchioles, are in place and the number of small air sacs, or alveoli, in which gaseous exchange takes place, are increasing. The next step in lung maturity is the production of surfactant, a very

thin film of which coats the air sacs. This substance reduces surface tension between molecules of fluid, allowing air to move in and out of the alveoli, which are able to remain inflated even after exhalation.

The lungs are the last of the major organs to form. They serve no purpose before birth because the fetus gets oxygen from its mother. Practice breathing (*see* page 71) during the last trimester occurs in bouts taking up 50 percent of the fetus' time, at various times of day but peaking in the hours of darkness. We are only just beginning to understand the brain mechanism that controls the on/off nature of fetal breathing. Things that will stop the baby breathing are a reduction in oxygen or glucose from the placenta, and the effects of drugs and alcohol. The lungs are maturing quickly between 30 and 35 weeks. Cortisol helps stimulate the production of surfactant.

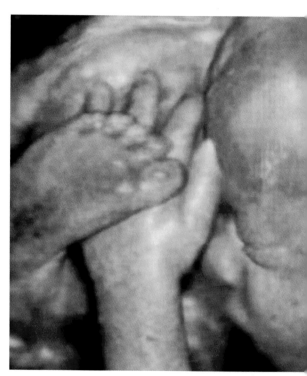

In the third trimester your baby is very well developed, as this 3-D scan shows, and does not have much room in the uterus.

SEX HORMONES

In boys and girls the adrenal glands continue to produce large quantities of an androgen-like hormone (DHEAS or Dehydroepiandrosterone sulfate) that is processed by enzymes in the liver before being passed to the placenta for conversion to estrogen. In boys the testes are producing testosterone, and some of this is converted by special target cells in the genitals to another male hormone that is essential for the development of external genitalia.

The testes descend from the back of the abdomen to the inside of the groin by 28 weeks, and to the scrotum by 32 weeks: they need to be there to complete maturation and for the start of sperm formation. Sperm cells can only mature in cooler temperatures, away from the warmth of the abdomen.

THE FINAL SPURT

From about 36 weeks the countdown to labor begins (*see* pages 110–13). Ninety-five percent of babies are now head-down, with their heads quite a way into the pelvic cavity. They usually gain 2.2lb (1kg) in this time, and will be laying down lots of fat. You will still feel movements, but they won't be as strong as they were because conditions in the uterus have become quite cramped. Your baby's heart beats now at a rate of 120–160 per minute, the digestive system is ready to receive liquids, and the fetal bone marrow is producing red blood cells.

The baby is now producing large quantities of cortisol in readiness for the moment when its own circulation takes over after delivery and it takes its first breath. The intestines are filling up with a dark green sticky substance called meconium, made up of dead skin cells and secretions from the baby's bowel, liver, and gall bladder. This is usually passed out of the baby's body in the first few days of life, but if it becomes stressed in the uterus, the baby may pass meconium, indicating that it needs to be born very soon.

HOW YOUR BODY IS CHANGING

Discomfort levels will be increasing now. You will only be able to breathe shallowly due to the size of your abdomen and the way it is restricting your diaphragm. You may have heartburn. As the weeks go by, the baby will engage or "drop" into your pelvis and your breathing should get easier, but then you will need to urinate more often because the baby is putting pressure on your bladder. You may have constipation and hemorrhoids.

A yellow, watery fluid, known as colostrum, may start leaking from your nipples. Your cervix may begin to thin out and open slightly. Your skin may feel tight and itchy and, even though you're feeling very tired, you may have difficulty sleeping.

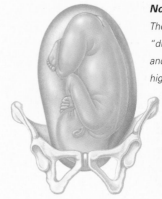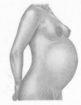

Not engaged
The baby has yet to "drop" into your pelvis and your bump remains high when in profile.

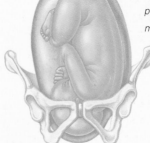

Engaged
Now the baby's head has descended into your pelvis, your bump is much lower than before.

windows of opportunity
your baby's brain

The brain is the most complex organ that will develop over the nine-month period; it is also the last to function properly. During pregnancy, you can have a significant impact on the development of this precious resource.

NEURAL STIMULATION

A baby is born with all the active brain cells it will ever have: no more will be produced. A newborn has two to three times as many brain cells as it will have by adulthood. At around eight months gestation, half the brain cells wither and die—this is a normal physiological process. In some cases it is because they have performed their vital function and are no longer needed; in others it is because they are superfluous and have not been stimulated

enough to make connections. At least 40 percent and possibly as many as 75 percent are lost during prenatal development.

As connections (synapses) between neurons are made, the stimulation of particular neural pathways triggers the release of neurotransmitters and special nerve growth factor that pass messages from one brain cell to another. This process helps secure greater numbers of brain cells into your baby's neural network. The number of brain cell

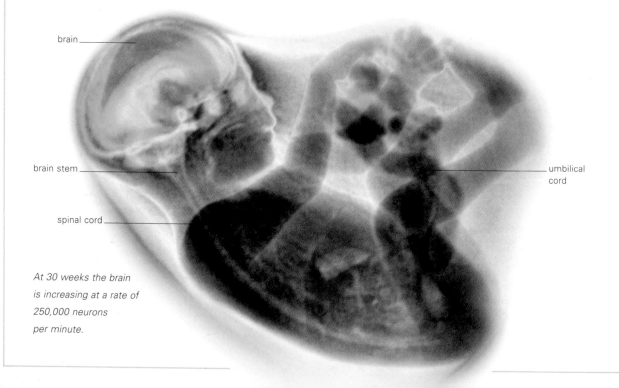

brain

brain stem

spinal cord

umbilical cord

At 30 weeks the brain is increasing at a rate of 250,000 neurons per minute.

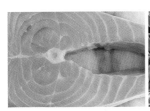 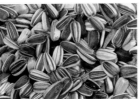

Oily fish and seeds are rich in essential fatty acids and are therefore great brain foods for the third trimester.

BRAIN DEVELOPMENT

27 weeks The surface of the brain is enlarging, but it still looks smooth. There is a growth spurt to increase the number of brain cells, develop dendrites (the projections from the cell body that receive impulses from other neurons), increase synaptic connections between brain cells, and develop the fatty myelin sheaths to protect the axons (projections carrying impulses away from the cell body). All of these processes require the laying down of fats, namely essential fatty acids.

30 weeks The surface of the brain has formed shallow, deeper grooves and convolutions, so it resembles a walnut. These undulations dramatically increase the surface area of the brain, so many more cells can be fitted in and connected up.

31 weeks Excess brain cells start to die off. This process of programmed cell death is designed to conserve useful neural pathways. It reaches a peak four weeks before birth. The neurons that die are deemed superfluous because they have not been adequately stimulated.

36 weeks The nervous system is fully developed and the brain has its full complement of 100 billion neurons.

connections will define your baby's intellectual potential so it is important to stimulate your baby while it is in the uterus (*see* pages 84–5).If your baby receives few stimulations, you reduce the number of connections or synapses as the cells are loosely wired and will die.

Your baby's environment is dependent on your environment and your behavior. Your baby can hear sound and see light; it is affected by your eating patterns; if you are in a Jacuzzi, the uterus warms up; if you exercise too vigorously, your baby may become short of oxygen. All these factors create sensory patterns and the development of your baby's brain is influenced by the nature of these inputs.

KEY BRAIN NUTRIENTS

Brain development requires different nutrients compared with other parts of the body—muscles and tissue need protein, for example; bones need minerals; but brain tissue needs fats. In fact, more than 60 percent of the human brain is composed of fats, in particular long-chain polyunsaturated fatty acids (LCPs).

Your baby cannot make its own fatty acids, so supplies must come from your stores or from fats in your diet. LCPs that are vital for the development of normal brain function in the last trimester include DHA (*see* page 21), which makes up 10–15 percent of the weight of the cerebral cortex (outer layer of the brain). Another important LCP is arachidonic acid (AA). Good food sources of this include seeds, such as sesame and pumpkin, and their oils, and oily fish (*see* page 135).

The placenta extracts the LCPs from the mother's blood and concentrates them in the baby's circulation, making them available to the developing brain. Brains that have low levels of LCPs available to them have significantly impaired development, lower intelligence, and may exhibit problems such as dyslexia. Firstborns are often more intelligent than their younger siblings because levels of DHA become depleted the more pregnancies you have.

If your diet is lacking in LCPs, your baby will most likely obtain the AA and DHA it requires from your brain. This may be one explanation for the poor concentration, poor memory, forgetfulness, and vagueness that many women find they experience later in pregnancy.

intelligence and gender

Your baby's intellectual development depends not only on the genes it inherits from you and your partner but also on its uterine environment and the stimulation it receives while there. Gender traits, on the other hand, follow a distinct male or female blueprint as the fetal brain develops.

WHAT IS INTELLIGENCE?

Intelligence depends on the number, arrangement, and interconnection of brain cells, and has three important aspects: the speed at which we can string thoughts together; our ability to learn; and our ability to problem-solve. Intelligence has many manifestations, including linguistic, mathematical, musical, visual, physical, and social.

Men have bigger brains than women and consequently more brain cells. Women compensate for their smaller brains by developing more complex connections between the different areas of the brain, so a woman's brain appears to have more areas of activity than a man's.

The emergence of gender differences

There are some marked differences in the types of intellectual behavior of male and female babies. In boys, once testosterone kicks in, it starts to play a part in the emergence of gender differences, in particular the development of the senses.

The effects of testosterone are far reaching, and gender differences are not just a matter of how large the brain is and how it's wired up. Girls and boys soon develop different specializations. Just a few hours after they are born, baby girls are more sensitive to touch than baby boys, and by a long way. Research has shown that tactile sensitivity in the fingers of even the most sensitive boys is less than that of the least sensitive girls.

Girls are also twice as sensitive to sound as boys, and they are therefore less tolerant of loud noise, becoming irritated and even anxious. Girls are more easily soothed by voices. They may be a long way off understanding language, but baby girls seem to be able to recognize that speech has an emotional aspect to it. Virtually from birth, they seem to be more interested than boys in communicating with other people, and will spend nearly twice as long maintaining eye contact with an adult, even if that person isn't talking to them.

Boys spend less time focusing on an adult, whether the adult is talking or not, which would suggest that they are more interested in their surroundings than in what they can hear.

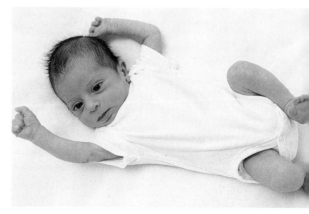

Baby boys tend to be awake for longer periods of time and are more active when they are awake than girls.

Baby girls love to gurgle at people, too. Most boys are equally happy to talk, but are just as content to talk to a cuddly toy in their crib or even an abstract geometric design on the wall. The natural inclination of girls to engage with others is illustrated by their ability, at just a few months old, to distinguish between photographs of people they know and those of strangers. Boys are unable to do this. Baby boys tend to be awake longer and are more active when they are awake than girls, indicative of the male brain being wired for activity.

BLUEPRINTS AND HORMONES

Hormones determine the distinct male or female organization of the brain as it develops in the uterus: the sexes share the same sexual identity

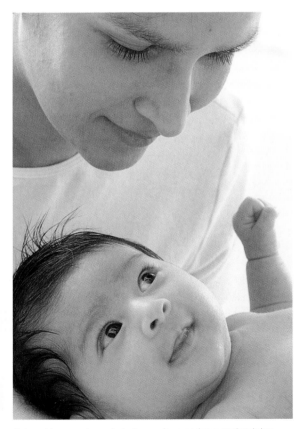

Baby girls spend nearly twice as long as boys maintaining eye contact with an adult, even if the adult isn't talking.

for only the first few weeks after conception. Thereafter, the genetic blueprint begins to unfold and their brains take on a distinctly male or female identity as they develop.

According to the XY (boy) blueprint, chromosomes initiate the development of testes. Around six weeks, a male fetus develops special cells that produce male hormones, or androgens, the most important of which is testosterone. These hormones stimulate the development of embryonic male genitalia, at the same time instructing the body not to develop any female sexual equipment. If the fetus has a female XX blueprint, the reproductive organs develop along female lines, without significant injections of male hormones.

The basic brain "template" of a fetus appears to be female, and, if a baby is going to be a girl, there is no intervention from male hormones as the embryonic brain develops. If an embryo is genetically male, however, radical hormonal involvement ensures that the brain develops along male lines. Boy babies are exposed to a massive dose of male hormones as their brains start to take shape.

Things can go wrong with this process, of course, just as they can with the development of any other part of the body. A male fetus may have enough male hormones to stimulate the formation of male sex organs, but not enough for the brain to develop according to a male pattern. Conversely, a female baby may be mistakenly exposed to male hormones and develop a male brain inside a female body.

Long-term effects

Throughout infant, teenage, and adult life, the way the brain is forged, along with the intricate interactions of hormones, will have a fundamental effect on the attitudes, behavior, and intellectual and emotional functioning of the individual. The way the brain takes shape affects how we see, smell, learn, think, feel, communicate, love, have sex, fight, succeed, or fail.

late pregnancy problems

The majority of pregnancies are straightforward, but, if problems do arise, it will help you to have some understanding of what is happening and why. Here are some of the more common complications that can occur in late pregnancy.

INTRAUTERINE GROWTH RESTRICTION (IUGR)

This describes the failure of a fetus to grow sufficiently, with the result that it weighs less than 5½lb (2.5kg) at term and is thinner and shorter than average. The condition is also known as fetal growth retardation, small for dates (or small for gestational age), or placental insufficiency.

Causes and symptoms

IUGR is usually the result of a fetal abnormality or undernourishment of the fetus, which may be caused by a placental problem, such as preeclampsia (*see* right); an infection such as rubella; or by the mother's lifestyle (smoking, drinking alcohol, drug abuse or inadequate diet). The condition is revealed by a smaller than normal uterus and ultrasound scan measurements of the fetus.

Risk to baby/management of condition

Small babies are at greater risk of infection, hypothermia, and low blood sugar, and may need monitoring in a special care baby unit after birth. Most will gain weight rapidly and reach a normal size.

PREECLAMPSIA

Also known as pregnancy-induced hypertension (PIH) or toxemia, preeclampsia affects up to eight percent of pregnancies, usually only mildly, and easily treated. It often happens in the second half of first pregnancies. You will be monitored for symptoms at every prenatal visit.

Causes and symptoms

The cause of preeclampsia is not fully understood but it may be an immune response by the mother. It runs in families, and is more common in younger and older mothers. You are also more likely to develop preeclampsia if you are overweight, have kidney disease or diabetes, or you already suffer from high blood pressure. High blood pressure is one of the main symptoms, along with fluid retention (edema) in the hands, feet, and legs and the presence of protein in the urine (because the kidneys aren't filtering properly). Symptoms usually develop gradually, but occasionally they can come on very quickly and may include headaches, blurred vision or flashing lights, vomiting, and pain in the upper abdomen. Contact your doctor immediately.

Risk to baby/management of condition

The only "cure" for this condition is delivery of the baby. If it is mild, bedrest at home may be recommended but with close monitoring of your blood pressure. If your blood pressure is moderately high, you will probably be admitted to the hospital to try to bring it down and to monitor the fetus more closely. If blood flow and the functioning of the placenta is affected, your baby will be at risk of IUGR (*see* left) or reduced oxygen supply. If you are beyond 36 weeks, induction is advisable.

Severe preeclampsia is life-threatening to both mother and baby. It may lead to eclampsia, which causes seizures and possibly

PLACENTA PREVIA

Placenta previa occurs when the placenta implants low down in the uterus. In some cases it may move upward as the uterus expands during the course of pregnancy but in others it covers part or all of the cervix. This happens in about 1 in 200 pregnancies, but is more common among older mothers. In marginal placenta previa, the placenta is low but only extends up to the edge of the cervix; complete placenta previa occurs when the cervix is completely covered.

Causes and symptoms

Placenta previa is more likely to happen if you have had several pregnancies, if the uterus has been scarred by previous surgery (for example, a cesarean delivery), or you have fibroids (a benign mass of muscle growing in the uterine wall). It is more common in multiple pregnancies.

There may be no symptoms, or there might be light to heavy vaginal bleeding from about week 24 onward. The condition is often picked up on the 20-week scan.

Risk to baby/management of condition

Follow-up scans will monitor the condition. If you have light bleeding, you may need only bedrest in the hospital. If placenta previa is complete, you will probably be admitted to the hospital around week 30 because of the risk of bleeding. There is an increased risk of postpartum hemorrhage (excessive loss of blood after delivery), so you may need to have a cesarean section even if the placenta previa is only marginal.

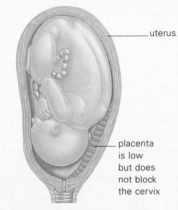
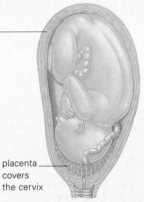
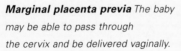

uterus

placenta is low but does not block the cervix

placenta covers the cervix

Marginal placenta previa *The baby may be able to pass through the cervix and be delivered vaginally.*

Complete placenta previa *A cesarean section is the safest option due to the high risk of hemorrhage.*

coma. You will be treated with anticonvulsants and drugs to lower your blood pressure and an emergency cesarean section is often necessary.

PLACENTAL ABRUPTION

The placenta does not usually come away from the wall of the uterus until after the baby is born, but sometimes (in about 1 in 120 pregnancies) part or all of it separates before delivery. Placental abruption is either

"revealed," in which case there is vaginal bleeding (in fact, this is the most common cause of bleeding beyond 28 weeks), or "concealed," when blood collects between the placenta and the uterine lining.

Causes and symptoms

The cause is unknown but there seems to be a link between placental abruption and chronic high blood pressure. The risk is greater if you smoke during

pregnancy, drink a lot of alcohol, or use recreational drugs. Placental abruption becomes more common as the number of pregnancies increases, if you have had one in a previous pregnancy, or if you suffer an abdominal injury during your pregnancy.

Symptoms can develop suddenly and, in addition to vaginal bleeding, which can be slight to very heavy, you may have abdominal cramps, constant intense abdominal pain, or backache. You may notice a reduction in fetal movement.

Risk to baby/management of condition

This condition can be life-threatening, especially for the fetus. If bleeding is heavy, you should go to the hospital immediately. If it is slight, your doctor will examine you internally, check the fetal heartbeat, and you may have a scan. A small abruption might just mean that you need bedrest (*see* page 87) in the hospital so the fetus can be monitored. If the pregnancy continues, the fetus may then be at risk of IUGR (*see* page 96). A large separation may mean you have to be induced or, if the situation is very serious, you may need to have an emergency cesarean section to save the baby.

PREMATURE RUPTURE OF MEMBRANES

The membranes enclosing the amniotic sac protecting the baby usually rupture just before labor or once it is under way, but in 1 in 14 women they break earlier.

Causes and symptoms

It isn't known exactly why this happens, but smoking seems to increase the risk. It is sometimes the result of infection spreading to the uterus from the vagina. The main symptom is a leak of amniotic fluid from the vagina:

either it may just be a trickle or it may be a flood.

Risk to baby/management of condition

If contractions don't start within a few hours or so, the baby will be at risk of infection. Also, a cord prolapse—when the cord drops into the cervix or vagina—may occur and restrict oxygen supply to the fetus if the head is not tightly up against the cervix. If you are 37 weeks into the pregnancy or more, then labor will probably start within a day or so; otherwise, you'll be induced. If you are less than 37 weeks, then you will probably stay in the hospital to be monitored for infection (and be treated if necessary) and fetal distress.

OBSTETRIC CHOLESTASIS

Itching is common in later pregnancy due to increased blood supply to the skin, but if it becomes severe—especially on the palms of your hands and soles of your feet—but there is no rash, it could be due to this rare but serious condition.

Causes and symptoms

Obstetric cholestasis is a liver disorder caused by bile salts being deposited under the skin. Reduced bile in the liver leads to a reduction in the absorption of vitamin K, needed for blood clotting. You may become jaundiced, your urine may be dark in color, and your stools pale.

Risk to baby/management of condition

The chances of bleeding are increased in both mother and baby. Treatment with ursodeoxycholic acid will reduce itching and restore liver function but you are likely to be induced at 37 or 38 weeks to reduce the risk of further complications.

CONGENITAL INFECTIONS

Most infections a woman may develop in pregnancy don't affect the fetus, but occasionally they cross the placenta. In late pregnancy, this may trigger premature labor or make the baby seriously ill at birth. It is also possible for the baby to pick up an infection as it passes through the birth canal.

• **Group B streptococcus (GBS)** Up to 20 percent of women have this bacterium in their vagina. They rarely show any symptoms but it can make a newborn very sick with pneumonia, a blood infection, or even, rarely, meningitis. Women are routinely screened during the last weeks of pregnancy and given antibiotics if they are carrying GBS.

• **Bacterial vaginosis** This is caused by an imbalance of vaginal bacteria and is often symptomless. It can lead to infection in the uterus and pelvic inflammatory disease. Women with BV are more likely to deliver prematurely and have babies with low birth weight because of reduced placental function.

• **Urinary tract infection** A quarter of women contract a urinary tract infection (UTI) during pregnancy because the flow of urine to the bladder slows. If you have a burning sensation when you urinate and pain near the bladder go to your doctor for antibiotics right away. If left, a serious infection might spread to the kidneys and blood, and would require intravenous antibiotic treatment in the hospital.

• **Chickenpox** Most women have had chickenpox or been vaccinated and are immune to the disease. However, if you haven't had it and you develop symptoms close to delivery, your baby may develop a severe infection (neonatal chickenpox). If this is the case, your baby will be given a special antibody injection at the time of delivery, which reduces the severity of the attack before symptoms appear.

OTHER CONDITIONS
See these pages for the following pregnancy conditions:
• premature labor, pages 114–15
• incompetent (weak) cervix, page 86
• too much amniotic fluid, page 86
• gestational diabetes, page 86
• problems with multiple pregnancies, pages 86–7
• miscarriage, pages 34–6

RHESUS INCOMPATIBILITY

The Rhesus (Rh) factor distinguishes blood types according to the presence or absence of certain proteins on the surface of red blood cells. As many as 85 percent of people have these proteins and are Rh positive; the rest don't and are Rh negative. Rhesus incompatibility describes a situation in which the mother's blood is Rh negative and her baby's blood is Rh positive.

Rhesus incompatibility doesn't usually present a problem in a first pregnancy because the mother's and the baby's bloodstreams do not mix. However, if

some of the baby's blood cells stray into the mother's circulation (during delivery, for example, or during amniocentesis), the mother may develop antibodies that would cross the placenta and attack an Rh-positive fetus in the future. This might cause severe anemia in the fetus in the uterus, heart failure, and jaundice once it was born.

If you are Rh negative, you will be offered injections (anti-D) during pregnancy and after delivery to destroy any Rh-positive cells you might have picked up and to prevent your body

from forming antibodies. Your blood will be routinely tested to see if antibodies have developed.

If antibodies are detected during a pregnancy, both you and your baby will need special care. You will have frequent blood tests and your baby will be checked for signs of anemia and heart failure. If antibody levels are low, the monitoring will continue to 38 weeks when you will be induced. If they are high, the baby may need blood transfusions (of Rh-negative blood) if it is too immature to be delivered.

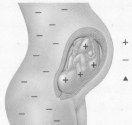

KEY:
+ Rh-positive blood
– Rh-negative blood
▲ Rh antibodies

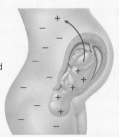

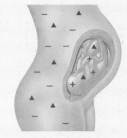

First pregnancy *for an Rh-negative mother with an Rh-positive baby. Their two bloodstreams don't mix.*

At delivery*, some of the baby's blood may leak into the maternal blood. The mother then develops Rh antibodies.*

In subsequent pregnancies*, Rh antibodies may cross the placenta and damage an Rh-positive baby's blood.*

good eating plan

Your diet is as important as ever: your growing baby is gaining weight many times faster than in early pregnancy. If your weight gain is inadequate or your diet is low in protein or calories, if you develop anemia, or if you are doing too much physical activity or working too hard, your baby's growth may be affected.

PROTEIN REQUIREMENTS

The requirement for protein is at an all-time high in the third trimester, since proteins are the building blocks for the generation of muscles and tissues. Proteins with different functions and capabilities are made from different combinations of amino acids. The amount of amino acids available to your baby from your bloodstream will be determined by your diet. However, your daily requirement of 2½oz (60g) of protein is also important for building up your own reserves as you prepare for labor, delivery, breastfeeding, and postpartum recovery (*see* pages 126–7).

Glycine

The amino acid glycine is now recognized as the driving force behind growth, playing a key role in the production of proteins. Your baby obtains glycine from your blood supply and from the placenta. Your intake of glycine comes from the protein in your diet (*see* page 134). The growing baby's demand for glycine is between 2 and 10 times greater than usual, and is also 2 to 10 times greater than the need for any other amino acid.

KEY NUTRIENTS FOR THE THIRD TRIMESTER

While a balanced diet is essential, there are some nutrients that play particularly important roles in your baby's development at this stage of pregnancy. For food sources *see* pages 134–7.

Choline

Choline is a phospholipid which is a "smart" fat found in the brain (*see* page 59). It is found in the myelin sheaths that insulate the axons, which carry nerve impulses from the cell bodies of nerve cells. Recent research has indicated that taking choline supplements may be beneficial. Rats were found to have developed vastly superior brains and had improved learning ability and better memory recall when given choline. The richest food source is egg yolks, but not all eggs are equal; buy organic eggs when possible.

Vitamin C

A lack of vitamin C has been linked to an increased risk of premature rupture of membranes (*see* page 98) and preterm labor. Vitamin C is needed to boost the immune system and protect against infection during the birth and help healing afterward. It aids the manufacture of collagen, connective tissue, and blood vessels for wound repair. It also improves the absorption of iron, stores of which need to be built up prior to labor.

Garlic

Garlic boosts circulation by dilating small arteries, improving circulation in the placenta, and decreasing the risk of blood clots. It reduces high blood pressure in pregnancy and boosts the immune system, protecting against infection.

Zinc

I believe that zinc has possibly the biggest role of all minerals in reproduction and pregnancy. It is important for growth: research has shown that babies born to mothers who took zinc supplements from the 19th week of pregnancy had a heavier birth weight and larger head circumference. A pregnant woman needs at least 20mg of zinc a day, but tends to get less than this from her diet. Check how much is supplied by your prenatal vitamin.

Lack of zinc is linked to pregnancy-related depression and postpartum depression. Research shows that women who consumed a lot of fish, which is rich in essential fats and zinc, during the last three months of pregnancy, were less likely to show symptoms of depression. Most zinc packs into the placenta at the end of pregnancy and it may be for this reason that many animals eat the after-birth. I am not advocating this—I merely observe that you don't hear of many cats or dogs being diagnosed with postpartum depression!

DHA

During the third trimester, the mother transfers to the fetus much of the DHA it needs for the development of its brain and nervous system (*see* pages 92–3). This has an effect on her own brain (she may lose as much as 3 percent of her brain

mass at this time!), so if you aren't already taking one, a supplement may be advisable. This also helps prevent postpartum depression and ensures an adequate supply for the nursing baby.

Vitamin K

Vitamin K plays a vital role in blood clotting: if there is a deficiency, bleeding can occur. In newborn babies this is called hemorrhagic disease, and it affects about 1 in 10,000 babies. It has therefore become standard practice to give vitamin K to newborns.

During the last trimester you should make sure that your diet includes foods rich in vitamin K, such as cauliflower, broccoli, and cabbage, so that you will pass vitamin K on to your baby in your milk. We get some of our vitamin K from bacteria living in the gut, which the baby does not have until colonization after it is born.

Iron

Eat lots of iron-rich foods to build up iron stores in the final trimester so that you have energy for labor; to protect against infection (by boosting your immune system); and to help prevent premature labor. It is important that you don't go into labor anemic, which could complicate labor and delivery. Up to 9oz (250g) of iron can be lost during delivery and up to twice this amount if you have to have a cesarean section.

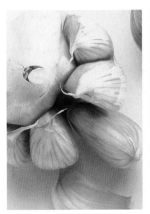
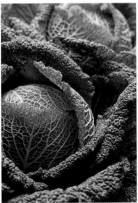

Third trimester nutrients: garlic boosts circulation in the placenta, while cabbage is a good source of vitamin K.

looking at lifestyle

As the third trimester advances, you'll be thinking more and more about the approaching labor and birth. Many women find it harder to sleep because they are getting bigger, so finding time to rest during the day is more important than ever.

EXERCISE IN THE THIRD TRIMESTER

You need a change of emphasis in your approach to exercise now. Think about building up your endurance so that you have stamina for labor. Exercise gently for 20 to 30 minutes every day: swimming, walking, yoga, and gentle stretching are all good.

You should also focus on key groups of muscles and joints ready for the birth. Squatting, for example, helps open up the pelvis, encourages the baby's head to engage, and improves the joints of the pelvis, knees, and ankles. It may be a good position for pushing when you are trying to deliver your baby.

As you gain more weight and your bump gets bigger, your center of gravity changes and you may find it more difficult to exercise. Research suggests, however, that women who exercise regularly improve their balance and have a better awareness of their center of gravity. They also tend to have a shorter labor and they are able to push their babies out more easily.

Make sure that your blood sugar level is balanced (*see* pages 16–17) and also keep an eye on how your baby reacts to you exercising. You should be able to feel it kick several times within the first 20 minutes after exercise. If it is in distress, its movement will be reduced to save energy. A lack of movement means it is not at all happy about you working out and you should try a different type of exercise—and discuss the situation with your obstetrician.

Exercise tips

• Don't strain and don't do too much exercise; this diverts blood flow away from the placenta.
• Always make sure you are well hydrated.
• Stop exercising immediately if you have any contractions, bleeding, or pain.
• Don't exercise if you have an infection (because that means you're under the weather) or if your baby is not growing well.

Toning your pelvic floor

Pelvic exercise is increasingly important from now on: you should do Kegel exercises every day. These involve tightening the ring of muscles that support the organs in the pelvic cavity and that get stretched and weakened during pregnancy. The urethra, vagina, and rectum pass through the pelvic floor. Draw the muscles up inside you as if you were trying to stop the flow of urine. Toning your pelvic floor will help your muscles stretch and recoil more easily and can prevent leaking of urine after the birth.

SEX AT THE END OF PREGNANCY

As you enter the final trimester, you may find your interest in sex waning again. Your large abdomen may make lovemaking physically challenging, and increased fatigue and back pain may also dampen your enthusiasm.

You can have sex well into your third trimester as long as the pregnancy is proceeding normally. Lying flat on your back may cause lightheadedness

"think about building up your endurance so you have the stamina for labor"

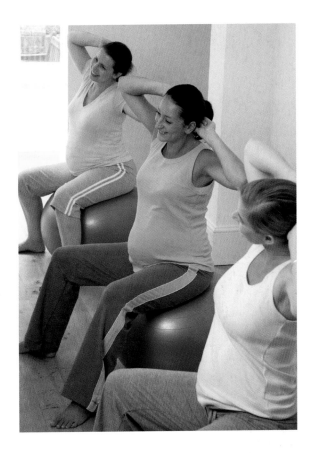

or nausea because your enlarged uterus is compressing the veins at the back of your abdomen, reducing your blood pressure. Orgasms can cause uterine contractions but, in a normal pregnancy, they won't lead to premature labor.

Later in pregnancy you may be advised to avoid intercourse if you develop problems such as vaginal bleeding, cervix or placenta irregularities (*see* pages 96–9), or there's risk of preterm labor.

If you've given birth prematurely before, you may need to be cautious. Also, if you're carrying two or more babies, your doctor may advise you to stop having intercourse a few weeks earlier than if you were expecting just one baby.

HYPNOBIRTHING

The philosophy behind hypnobirthing builds on the principles of natural childbirth: that the more relaxed you are during labor, the less pain you will feel. You will also have greater control over your body and the outcome for mother and baby is likely to be safer and more comfortable.

Fear of pain or of the birth experience leads to tense muscles and anxiety, which may complicate the birth. Armed with knowledge and well-practiced relaxation techniques you are better equipped to follow your natural birthing instincts. This doesn't mean that you give birth in a trance, but rather a relaxed state of focused concentration that enables communication with the subconscious. This allows the control of pain and encourages the release of endorphins to replace the stress hormones that create pain.

With a birthing partner, you will learn:
- self-hypnosis and relaxation techniques to build confidence and instill calm at each stage of labor
- positions for greater comfort during labor and birth
- visualization, breathing, and massage techniques
- the neuromuscular workings of the body
- methods of releasing fear and tension.

You may be able to teach yourself self-hypnosis.

Hypnobirthing supporters claim that its methods reduce the need for pain-killing drugs; shorten the first stage of labor; eliminate fatigue during labor, leaving the mother with energy for the birth; reduce the risk of complications and hence intervention; produce good-tempered babies and less-stressed parents; and aid faster postpartum recovery.

bonding before birth

Most women sense the importance of slowing down mentally and physically in the last few weeks of their pregnancy. This is prompted by anticipation of the birth and the physical need to rest because they're getting increasingly tired and their bodies are telling them that they need to ease up.

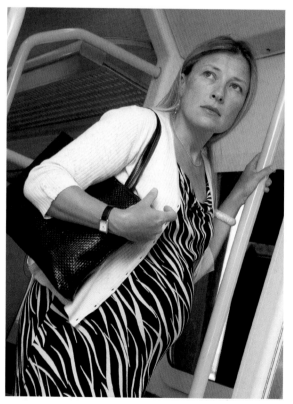

"you need time to prepare emotionally –give up work early"

COMMUNICATION CHANNELS

Much is written about bonding and emotional attachment between mother and baby after the birth but, now that we know how receptive the fetus is when it comes into the world (*see* pages 84–5), we can see this as a continuation of connections made before birth. During the last three months of pregnancy, your baby is mature enough physically and intellectually to send and receive sophisticated messages. You set the pace, provide the cues, and mold your baby's responses. Keep the channels open with lots of reassuring messages and your baby will continue to thrive.

It is important to be emotionally strong, prepared, and ready for birth. Women under emotional stress during pregnancy tend to have babies who cry excessively and who are irritable by nature. Consider how sensitive we are to emotions expressed by those around us: we experience both positive and negative feedback on a daily basis. It is the same for babies during their last weeks in the uterus, when they are more wakeful and alert to their surroundings: they receive chemical signals transmitted by your positive and negative emotions.

HORMONAL LINKS

Prenatal research leads us to believe that there is a connection between what a mother thinks and feels and her baby via hormones. There is also a link between the mother's emotional life during

BONDING CHECKLIST

- Babies can hear—make sure yours has plenty to listen to.
- Babies can learn—help yours make associations between the sensations it experiences.
- Babies can have attitude—send positive thoughts and feelings via your hormones.
- Babies know how to chill—relax and your baby will relax with you.
- Babies have a personality—it will be molded by their experiences.
- Babies want to be with their mothers— do whatever you can to give your baby the best emotional start in life.

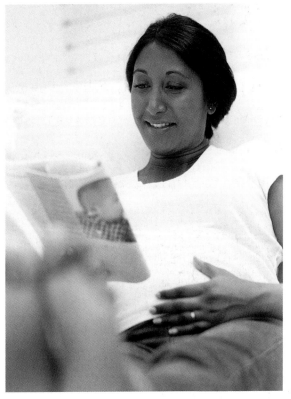

Spend time before the birth focusing on the imminent arrival and thinking about what it will mean to be a mother.

pregnancy and the later personality of her child. Short-term emotional upsets that are quickly resolved do not harm the baby, but major emotional strife and unresolved stress may result in emotionally troubled children.

Blood flow is certainly adversely affected by stress and is improved by the use of relaxation techniques. The babies of depressed women tend to have a higher heart rate and remain in a heightened state of arousal in response to stress, apparently unable to inhibit their response. Those regularly subjected to negative maternal mood are also likely to be smaller at birth. So, it is important to be aware of your emotional input into your baby as well as meeting its physical needs.

EMOTIONAL PREPARATION

You need time to prepare emotionally before the birth, which is why I encourage women to give up work early. Take time to think about how you are going to be as a mother. We know that the early days and weeks after the birth are important for the baby's emotional health and development. You can read books, follow programs, and check out every pregnancy and childbirth guru there is, but in those early days, you are the person who understands your baby best. You will work out for yourself your baby's best interests.

The only way to do this is to spend time together. So much time goes into the material trappings of preparing the nursery and reestablishing normal daily life after the birth. When I look back to the time I had my children, I wish I had appreciated how important these early days were to the emotional health of both of us. I would have been far less preoccupied with the chores and minutiae of daily life.

Focus on making room for this baby in your life: no prenatal classes can prepare you for the days and weeks ahead. Yes, babies need feeding and changing, but all a baby really wants to do is be with its mother. Accept a pearl of wisdom from someone who has been there: forget everything else for the first couple of weeks and it will pay dividends. Use your time now to sort out ways of achieving this.

expecting more than one

If you are expecting more than one baby, every day counts now. Each week that passes with your babies remaining safely inside your uterus, the better it is for their growth and development, so every attempt will be made to keep them there.

ENSURING WELL-BEING

You and your babies will be closely monitored because a multiple pregnancy is considered higher risk, and your delivery date will be under constant review. Your blood pressure will be checked regularly to make sure there are no signs of preeclampsia (*see* page 96), and regular ultrasound scans will monitor your babies' individual growth and also any growth difference between them, which may indicate problems (*see* pages 86–7). You may also be advised to have tests that check fetal well-being, such as a nonstress test (*see* facing page). You will be taught to be alert to your babies' movements.

PRETERM LABOR

The most frequently encountered problem with a multiple pregnancy is prematurity. We don't know precisely why labor starts in a single pregnancy, so the causes of premature labor with twins (or more) are similarly speculative.

Because the uterus is so distended it may send signals or respond to hormonal triggers that initiate contractions prematurely. The amniotic membranes may rupture too early. We do know that the fetus plays a part in the initiation of labor, so if two or more babies are present, perhaps together they are responsible for a greater stimulus.

Any pregnancy is considered full term by 38 weeks. Although singletons may be induced by 42 weeks, twins are usually considered for induction by 40 weeks. Proceeding any further with the pregnancy increases the risk of intrauterine death

of a baby. Also, the mother is at increasing risk of placental abruption, hemorrhage, and high blood pressure. Twins sharing a placenta and amniotic sac are at a higher risk of cord entanglement and twin-to-twin transfusion. Delivery may be encouraged as early as 34 weeks in order to avoid complications.

The increased number of multiple pregnancies is partly the result of assisted reproductive techniques. The pregnancies that result are likely to be closely monitored and the result may be earlier delivery. Fear of litigation may also be driving preterm intervention as well as the predominance of cesarean section deliveries of twins and multiples.

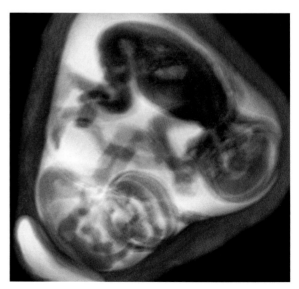

This MRI scan is of 32-week-old twin boys. The babies share a placenta (lower left, in pink) and amniotic sac.

VAGINAL DELIVERY OR CESAREAN SECTION

If you go into premature labor, you may be able to deliver vaginally since labor progresses very quickly. But the majority of multiples are born by cesarean section because it is considered safer for the babies. The most common reasons are because of the babies' positions or concern about the delivery of the second twin. There is little way of knowing how the birth of a second twin will progress until the first has been delivered.

If the first baby is head-down, however, doctors will usually perform a vaginal delivery, and some of them will try to deliver the second baby in the same way, even if it is breech, but this will depend on the skill of the doctor and the size of the baby. It is also possible, by a procedure known as external version, to maneuver the breech baby around in the uterus before birth.

If a vaginal delivery is planned, you may be advised to have an epidural so that an emergency cesarean could be carried out if needed without delay. Fetal monitoring will be continuous during labor, and delivery of the second twin within half an hour of the first is desirable. Contractions may weaken after the first delivery and you may be given pitocin to help things along.

When a cesarean section is necessary

You may need a cesarean for one of the same reasons that would apply to any other pregnant woman: if there's a problem with labor; the babies don't fit through the birth canal; there's fetal distress; or if the babies are in danger because of severe pregnancy-induced hypertension or a placental abruption (*see* pages 97–8). All of these are more common if you're carrying two or more babies.

If your twins are locked in a position in which neither of them can move, they will have to be delivered by cesarean section, as will all triplets and higher multiples. Also, if one or more of your babies are breech, you are more likely to have a cesarean.

WHAT IS A NONSTRESS TEST?

This measures fetal heart rate while the mother is at rest and the baby (or babies) is moving. It followed research showing that if a baby is not getting enough oxygen, its heartbeat will not show as much "variability." What this means is that the heartbeat remains constant despite, for example, the baby moving about. Normally, the heart rate fluctuates with movement, and when it doesn't it is taken as a sign of stress.

A fetal monitor is attached to the mother's abdomen and records the baby's movements and the response of its heart. The test is said to be "reactive" if the heart rate gets faster by at least 15 beats as the baby moves, twice in a 20-minute period. The test is described as "nonreactive" if the heart shows no speeding up during a 40-minute period.

A baby's heart rate is a good indicator of its well-being and this test can be reassuring for an expectant mother.

STRIVING FOR 40 WEEKS

Work toward a delivery date as close to 40 weeks as possible. Be especially conscious of your diet at this time to ensure that each twin is getting the nutrients it needs. A good all-round multivitamin and mineral supplement should contain vitamins C and E, folic acid, zinc, and iron.

Increase your intake of all fluids, especially water. Dehydration and a reduction of amniotic fluid are both contributing factors in preterm labor. The uterus is a muscle and will contract when dehydrated. If contractions do start, drink at least two large glasses of water or juice and lie on your side for at least half an hour to increase blood flow to the uterus. Then, if you're still getting them, call your doctor or midwife.

Increase the amount of bedrest or relaxation after the 28th week. It's a good idea to take as much pressure off the uterus as possible. Enjoy frequent naps, and do things sitting or lying down whenever possible. Lie on your side to take weight off the babies and off the back of your abdomen, where the largest blood vessels are located.

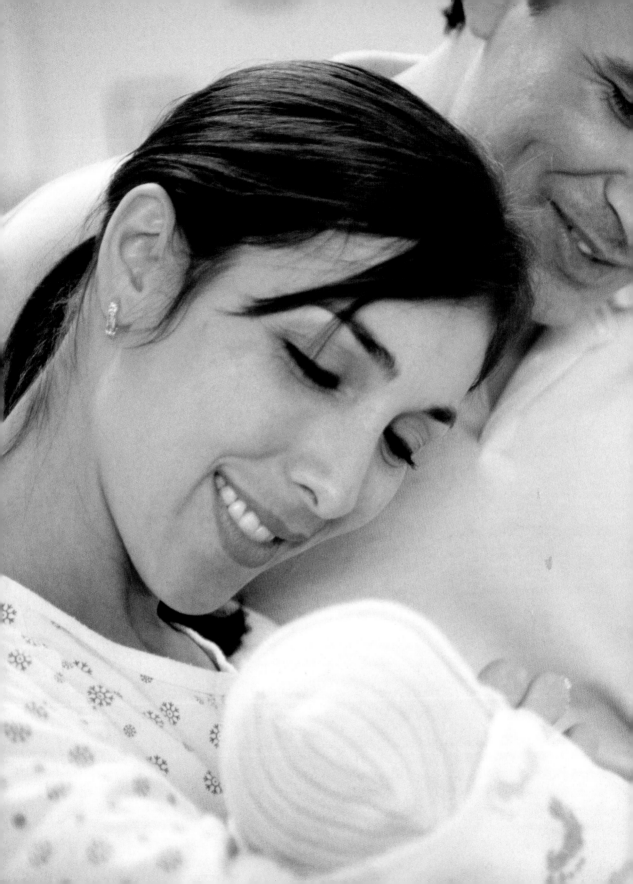

LABOR, BIRTH & BEYOND

At last the moment when you will meet your baby is imminent, but the process of giving birth can be exhausting and draining for both you and your baby. This chapter helps you prepare your body and mind as the countdown to labor begins. And after the birth an all-round recovery program is essential. Here you will find my recommendations, including plenty of rest and good nutrition, to help you cope with the first few weeks of motherhood.

preparing for labor

Going through labor has been compared to running a marathon: if you are prepared physically and mentally, you will get through it all the more easily. Not all labors are predictable, and to cope you will need determination, energy, stamina—and a good coach.

THE RIGHT MINDSET

Mindset has a huge part to play. Having looked after hundreds of women in labor, I know that how you feel during delivery has an enormous influence on how you deliver. If you are relaxed and confident, the outcome will usually be good. If you are wracked with fear and fatigue, labor will be slower. A study in Michigan found that anxious women labored longer than calm women. It's also important to have an open mind: flexibility is the key.

There are endless books on the subject and many ways of preparing for labor, but on the day, a good physician or midwife counts for everything. Being able to trust and feeling safe and secure with your provider are vital to the process. His or her familiarity with patterns of behavior at each stage of labor will give you a better understanding of what is happening to your body and how to cope.

Taking time to think

A lot of women work late into their pregnancies and don't have much time for mental preparation, but planning ahead is really important. As a couple, you should really savor the last couple of weeks together before the birth. You may be impatient to have your baby, but it will be a long time before you have time alone together like this again. Start to plan now for how you will share responsibility once the baby is here.

BUILDING UP RESERVES

In the final weeks, rest is crucial. You need to build up your energy reserves for labor. You are not likely to be sleeping as well toward the end, because it may be difficult to get comfortable. So, put your feet up at any time throughout the day, practice deep breathing to relax and improve blood flow to the placenta, and communicate and bond with your baby.

FOODS FOR LABOR

● One of your most important aims in preparing to give birth should be to build up energy reserves. This means stocking up on complex carbohydrates so that glycogen stores in the liver and muscles (for helping muscles contract) are increased. Complex carbohydrates will also help keep blood-sugar levels stable, maintaining energy.

● You will need vitamins and minerals to facilitate the conversion of glucose into energy. Those required include B vitamins, choline, vitamin C, iron, calcium, magnesium, chromium, and coenzyme Q_{10}. You will also need vitamin K for blood clotting and zinc for hormone production and healing after the birth.

● If your stomach feels restricted at this stage you may prefer to eat smaller meals more frequently throughout the day. Snacks are very important to maintain energy supplies, build up energy reserves, and during labor itself.

● Your energy levels will be affected if you become dehydrated. So, maintain your fluid intake at all times.

COUNTDOWN TO LABOR

In the time before your due date, you'll feel more confident if you're taking positive steps toward preparing for labor and birth and planning for looking after your baby after its arrival.

34 weeks

You will have started prenatal or active birth classes and will be learning techniques to help cope with the birth. Visualize your baby and communicate with it. Start massaging your perineum with oil to increase its flexibility and stretchiness ready for the birth. Stock up on iron-rich foods.

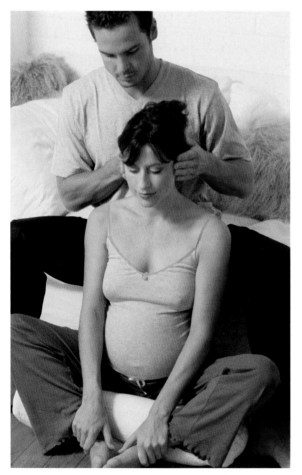

Savor time spent just with your partner before the two of you become three. Plan together for when the baby arrives.

35 weeks

Exercise gently for a little while every day, and don't forget to keep doing your Kegel exercises (*see* pages 102–3).

36 weeks

You may be feeling pretty fed up with being pregnant by now. You will be especially tired if you're sleeping badly because you're uncomfortable when lying down. Consider a relaxing aromatherapy massage. Start stretching exercises designed to strengthen the pelvic area, such as tailor sitting (sitting with your knees apart and feet together). This can be one of the most comfortable ways to sit during pregnancy and is also a great way of releasing tension in the lower back. Also practice positions for labor, such as squatting or kneeling.

37 weeks

Labor could happen any day now and you're probably starting to feel anxious. Keep practicing your relaxation techniques. Rest is more important than ever. Take vitamin C and zinc (check your prenatal supplement); both are necessary for hormone production in preparation for delivery.

38 weeks

Start to build up your carbohydrate intakes. Stock up on magnesium- and calcium-rich foods for good muscle contractions in labor.

39 weeks

Coenzyme Q_{10} improves the cells' ability to use oxygen and is used by athletes to maximize their performance: make sure your diet includes rich food sources. Also eat foods rich in vitamin K, which is vital for blood clotting.

40 weeks

Delivery should be any day now. Rest whenever you can and practice relaxation techniques as well as good positions for labor.

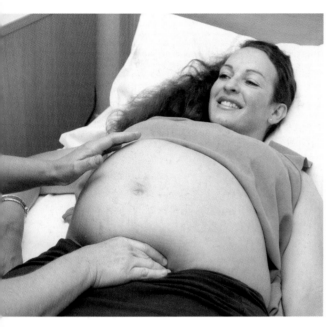

"the best position for your baby when you go into labor is an anterior position"

BABY'S BEST POSITION FOR BIRTH

The best position for the baby to be in when you go into labor is head down, with the back of its head toward the front of your pelvis. This is described as an anterior position, and labor is nearly always shorter and easier as a result.

Some babies go down into the pelvis with the back of their head toward their mother's spine. This position is described as posterior and is more likely to lead to:
• a longer labor
• backache for you both during and between contractions
• labor being slower
• a greater chance of getting tired, since it may take longer for the head to rotate.

Posterior presentation labor can be very uncomfortable because the baby's head is so close to your spine. The best position for you in labor might be on all fours because this helps the baby drop away from your spine.

Western women are more likely to have posterior babies than women who work in traditional ways in fields or bending over cooking pots. This is because, if you're sitting in a car, or on the sofa watching television, or working at a computer, your pelvis is tipped backward. In this

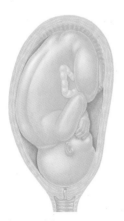

Anterior position—the back of the baby's head is toward the front of the mother's abdomen.

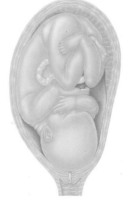

Posterior position—the back of the baby's head is toward the mother's spine.

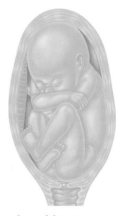

Breech position—the baby is not positioned head down; rather its buttocks are the presenting part.

position, the heaviest part of your baby, the back of the head and the spine, will tend to swing around to the back. But if your life involves a lot of upright activities, your pelvis is always tipped forward and your baby is more likely to go down into the pelvis in an anterior position.

BREECH POSITION

If your baby is in the breech position, it means that its bottom, not the head, is down in the pelvis ready to come out first. At 28 weeks some 25 percent of all babies are breech. The majority of these will turn during the third trimester, and less than 4 percent of all babies are breech at term. If the baby doesn't turn, you will probably need to have a cesarean section.

HELPING YOUR BABY INTO POSITION

Optimal fetal positioning is all about encouraging your baby to take up an anterior position.
• Sit on a cushion in the car to lift your bottom up.
• Make sure your favorite chair doesn't make your bottom go down and your knees come up.
• Take regular breaks and move around if your job involves a lot of sitting.
• Scrub the floors! When you're on all fours, the back of your baby's head swings to the front of your abdomen.
• Watch television on all fours—you may find you can tolerate this position for only 10 minutes or so.

Many experienced midwives are convinced that the mother's posture during late pregnancy does affect the position of her baby. Posture affects the interior shape of the uterus over time. Standing with more weight on one foot than the other or crossing your legs can shift or twist the uterus by shortening supportive ligaments on one side. It is therefore possible that you may be able to influence the position of your baby with your own body movements and position. Slow pelvic rocking on your hands and knees from 37 weeks onward may be beneficial, although research is inconclusive.

INDUCTION

Induction is a deliberate attempt to start labor by artificial means. Most women prefer to go into labor naturally, but in certain circumstances the risk of continuing a pregnancy is greater than the potential risk of intervention.

Reasons for induction

Induction carries a risk so it should only be advised for the following medical reasons:
• The baby has gone more than a week beyond term. Hospital policy varies on this, but the danger is that the placenta will start to fail.
• Raised blood pressure. The decision to induce will depend on the severity of the condition, the level of protein in your urine, and the maturity of the baby.
• Diabetes in the mother can put the fetus at risk in late pregnancy. It will lead to a bigger baby so induction or a cesarean section may be recommended.
• Early rupture of membranes. Some hospitals recommend induction, while others check that there is no cord prolapse and send you home to wait for spontaneous labor.
• Poor obstetric history—previous stillbirths, babies with abnormalities, or conditions such as placental abruption.

Methods of induction

• Sweeping a finger across the membranes. Your midwife or doctor can do this as part of a vaginal examination. It may be sufficient to start labor if your due date is close.
• Prostaglandin gel pessaries are inserted into the vagina, or gel is applied to the cervix to help soften and ripen the cervix and stimulate contractions.
• Intravenous oxytocin drip to initiate contractions.

Natural alternatives

In most cases, you will be given several days' notice of induction, which gives you an opportunity to try natural alternatives, such as acupuncture, homeopathic remedies, reflexology, and cranial osteopathy. However, these should be attempted only if you are healthy, your pregnancy has been free of complications, and you have reached your due date. Always consult a qualified practitioner.

premature labor

Prematurity is defined as being born before 37 weeks gestation. These babies represent 10 percent of all births, and although they account for 50 percent of long-term handicaps, many do catch up and progress just as well as full-term babies.

DANGERS OF PREMATURE BIRTH

The elements of a fetus' life-support system develop at different rates in the uterus, but they are all scheduled to be on line from the end of 40 weeks, ready for birth and separation from the placenta. One of the greatest threats to a baby's well-being is coming out of an environment that is safe before it has had time to prepare.

Premature babies do not yet have fully developed lungs or kidneys, and there can be long-term consequences for their health if these organs are not ready at birth. The brain is still organizing itself rapidly, and many problems arising from prematurity are to do with neural development.

WHY IT HAPPENS

Premature labor occurs when uterine contractions start too early. Throughout the last trimester of pregnancy, women experience gentle tightenings of the uterus: Braxton Hicks "practice" contractions. For some reason, with premature labor, these contractions grow stronger, and you are likely to become fully dilated very quickly.

Premature labor may be caused by an infection of the urinary tract or the vagina; stress; heavy work; or nutritional factors. In some women the cervix shortens during pregnancy and it is thought that half of these cases may result in premature birth. In addition, the risk of premature birth is increased by smoking, alcohol and drug abuse; previous premature labor; or certain long-term health problems such as diabetes. There is also a link between gum disease and premature labor (*see* below).

Stressed fetuses pump steroids out of their adrenal glands, which is also thought to be one of the triggers for labor at term. The steroids may be the baby's signal to accelerate preparations for delivery because things are getting difficult in the uterus. Recent Australian research showed that a baby monitors food resources available in the uterus and if they become depleted, it sends a "let's get on with it" signal.

Maternal stress prompts the mother's adrenal glands in the same way. If the mother is under

PREMATURE LABOR AND GUM DISEASE

Recent studies have shown that women with gum disease have a six times greater risk of going into premature labor than women with healthy gums. Bacteria migrate from the gums in the bloodstream and seem to specifically target the placenta and amniotic fluid. Smoking increases the risk of premature labor anyway (by 25 percent) but it also makes gum disease more likely because it reduces resistance to bacteria in the mouth. It is thought that, since pregnancy challenges the immune system, women may have a harder time keeping in check bacteria normally present in the mouth. It's therefore advisable to maintain good oral hygiene throughout pregnancy.

stress, her increased hormone production may cause estrogen levels to rise sooner than they should, and trigger labor.

PREVENTION

Sometimes premature labor can be halted by drugs that stop the contractions. You will have total bedrest and the baby will be monitored for fetal distress. If labor cannot be stopped, it might at least be possible to postpone it for a few days so that you can be given corticosteroid injections to improve the maturity of the fetal lungs. Steroids will also encourage the deposition of brown fat, which enables body heat to be retained. Newborn babies are not good at regulating their body temperature in the best of circumstances, and premature babies have even more of a problem.

The number one rule in preventing prematurity is to combat stress. Get plenty of rest. Make sure your diet is nutritionally balanced and stay well hydrated. Your blood volume needs to be good to carry large amounts of nutrients. There is also evidence that extra vitamin C reduces the risk of premature rupture of membranes.

PREMATURE DELIVERY

Many premature babies are delivered by cesarean section (*see* page 123) because the monitoring is not reassuring. When mothers deliver vaginally,

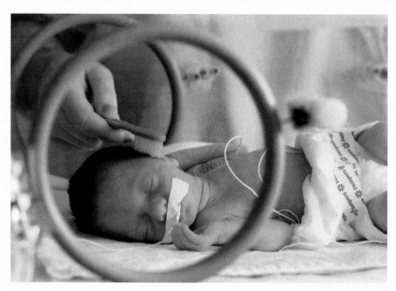

Preterm babies who are stroked and cuddled gain weight more quickly than those who aren't touched, and are often able to go home sooner as a result.

labor may be faster because premature babies are smaller and the cervix does not always have to be fully dilated for the baby to pass through. However, the baby is less likely to be in the ideal position for birth—head down—another reason that delivery by cesarean section is more likely.

THE NEONATAL INTENSIVE CARE UNIT (NICU)

If you are in labor prematurely, you may be transferred to a hospital with a high risk obstetric unit and a neonatal intensive care unit. After the birth, your first visit to the intensive care unit may be daunting. It can be upsetting to see your tiny baby being fed by tube, with wires attached to all parts of his body. The equipment will seem less

alarming, however, once you understand what it does.
• Ventilators help your baby breathe.
• Incubators help regulate body temperature.
• Your baby will probably be fed intravenously, perhaps with a drip, syringe pump, or infusion pump, because he can't suck or tolerate normal food.
• Monitoring equipment enables staff to check his heart rate, breathing patterns, and blood-glucose levels.

Babies who are stroked and cuddled grow and develop more quickly. Studies of preterm babies of less than 36 weeks show that touching increases their weight gain, enabling them to go home earlier. The need for touch cannot be overemphasized (*see* pages 121–3).

impact of labor

After nine months in the uterus, your baby is aware of its surroundings and sensations are a major part of its life. But birth comes as a shock: one minute your baby is floating blissfully in warm fluid, the next it is thrust into the birth canal.

A DIFFICULT JOURNEY

It is now thought that the fetus determines when pregnancy is over and labor should begin. It might be triggered by hunger and a rise in cortisol levels. Your baby's epinephrine levels and heartbeat will reach their highest ever, and the surge in stress hormones increases blood flow to the heart, lungs, and brain in preparation for birth.

The short journey down the birth canal is a dangerous one and your baby has to make complicated adjustments to its life-support system in order to be able to breathe. Once in the outside world, delay isn't an option.

Speaking as a midwife, childbirth is the most amazing experience. Understanding what is happening to your body, feeling safe and secure and having confidence in the process, being focused, and feeling in control are crucial. Many women think that the best birth is one without drugs. To me, it's one without preconceived ideas. If you need drugs, you need them; you'll have a constant dialog with your doctor or midwife, and it's fine to change your mind about decisions you made before labor.

Coping with labor is about managing stress and pain. The body releases more endorphins as the pain builds. They alter your perception of pain, making you feel nice and floaty. If you get anxious and tense, you'll release epinephrine, which counteracts the effects of the endorphins:

WATER BIRTH

Immersion in warm water relieves pain and aids relaxation, releasing tension and making it easier to go with the flow of contractions. The water supports you, making it easier to try different positions. Inhalation analgesia might be available during a water birth, and the baby can be monitored. It is a low-tech way of conducting labor and leads to fewer interventions, but little research has been done to identify potential risks. Some doctors and midwives prefer you to be out of the pool for delivery.

A water birth is not considered suitable if the birth becomes complicated. This might be the case if you're expecting more than one baby; your baby is breech; or you have mild preeclampsia (*see* page 96). Water birth might not be advisable if either you or your baby need treatment; it has been more than 24 hours since your water broke; you have been induced; you've had sedative drugs or an epidural; your labor is premature; or you've experienced recent bleeding.

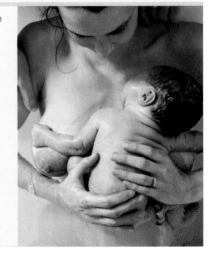

stress hormones slow down labor and make you feel more pain. So, stress relief and pain relief are interlinked.

PATTERNS OF BEHAVIOR IN LABOR

Experienced labor floor personnel can often tell how dilated a woman in labor is by the sounds she makes. In early labor (0–4 cm dilation), a woman is usually up and around, chatting to all around her, and excited about contractions. Take advantage of gravity and stay upright if you can. This will encourage the head to descend into the cervix, which will help it dilate. I encourage women to use a TENS machine during this stage (*see* page 119).

Once labor is established (5–8cm), women become more passive, concentrating on their breathing and relaxation techniques, and they don't appreciate interruption. Massage to the lower back can bring relief during this phase and will encourage the release of endorphins. If you're having a water birth you'll be allowed into the water at this time (*see* box opposite).

EATING AND DRINKING DURING LABOR

I am a great believer in eating while you're in labor, although this may not be allowed in some hospitals. You need energy, and in early labor you're still active and able to eat. Be guided by what appeals to you. Meat and other high-fat foods may be too heavy for the digestive system. Complex carbohydrates are good because they provide a steady release of energy to help you work through the contractions. Choose from bread, cereals, pasta, potatoes, and bananas. Sugary foods are easy to eat and a treat. They give you an energy boost, but the energy quickly dissipates, so avoid too much chocolate or sweet drinks.

Eat only as much as is comfortable. Eat regularly: a snack every hour or so in early labor will store energy for the hours ahead. Later on, you may find that you do not want to eat much.

Labor is thirsty work and delivery rooms can be hot. So you will certainly want plenty of water.

WHAT IS FETAL DISTRESS?

A baby who is doing well during labor will have a strong, stable heart rate and will respond to a stimulus. When you are having a contraction, there may be pressure on the baby and its heart rate will decrease. This is a normal adaptation and will show on a monitor. If the heart rate does not speed up again at the end of the contraction, however, it might mean the baby is tiring or its oxygen supply has been compromised.

If a baby is not tolerating labor well, the condition is described as "fetal distress." It is serious and demands immediate action. A baby in distress may also pass its first stool (meconium). Your doctor's approach to meconium will depend on how it looks. If it is thick, green, and grainy, and it is accompanied by a reduction in heart rate, an emergency cesarean section will be recommended.

Fetal distress may occur before the onset of labor, for example because the amniotic fluid is low and the baby has stopped growing. It may be detected during a scan or a nonstress test (*see* page 107). Labor may then be induced or a cesarean section performed.

Don't worry about needing to go to the toilet frequently: it's an excellent way of keeping mobile and encouraging the baby's head to descend.

Opinion is divided about drinking isotonic drinks used by athletes. They are designed to be quickly absorbed and provide energy for vigorous exercise. Some doctors recommend them, some don't. You may wish to avoid carbonated sodas and acidic fruit juices because they might make you feel sick.

The reason why women were routinely starved in labor in the past was because of concern over the possibility of needing a general anesthetic for a cesarean section. There is a small risk that food might be regurgitated and inhaled as the anesthetic takes effect. In fact, this risk is almost nonexistent if good anesthetic practice is followed, and most cesarean sections these days are carried out using spinal anesthesia or an epidural.

DIFFICULT BIRTHS

One in ten births can be described as difficult and traumatic for mother and baby and may have after effects on both. A difficult birth experience can leave you feeling depressed and vulnerable, which may take some time to get over (*see* page 122).

As the baby travels down the birth canal, its head—the widest part of its body—molds because the bones of the skull have not yet fused. The overall effect is to compress the head. In most cases, it recovers in a matter of days, but occasionally the bones remain locked together and growth and development of skull and brain can be affected. The compressive forces at play during birth often feed into the spine and pelvis, resulting in a greater tension and less freedom of movement in certain joints. This may have long-term consequences for the health and well-being of a developing child. Many common conditions during infancy are thought to have their origins in what is known as unresolved cranial molding: difficulties with feeding and sleeping, constant crying, colic, ear problems, and visual disturbances.

Assisted delivery may have similar long-term side effects. The use of forceps and vacuum extraction often increases cranial molding, body tension, and shock in a baby. If you have had a vacuum or forceps delivery, your baby may cry a lot in the early days. Cranial osteopathy, in which a specialized practitioner gently manipulates the cranial and spinal bones, works well for babies

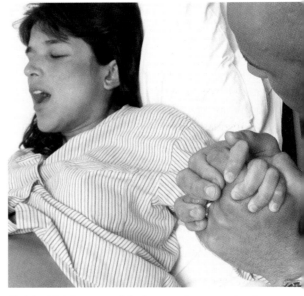

If giving birth becomes difficult, try to focus on relaxation techniques and allow your birth partner to support you.

and small children who develop problems such as sleeplessness that may have resulted from a difficult birth experience.

Babies born vaginally have longer to prepare for birth, both physiologically and psychologically, as they pass through the birth canal. Babies born by cesarean section, on the other hand, have to adjust in a short space of time as they hurriedly enter the outside world and may initially have more respiratory problems because amniotic fluid in the lungs doesn't get squeezed out by the birth canal.

THE EFFECTS OF PAINKILLING DRUGS ON YOUR BABY

● Opiate drugs, such as demerol, given for pain relief during labor, cross the placenta. There has been much debate about whether their use is detrimental to the baby.

● The use of excess doses of pain-relief medication has been linked in Swedish studies to babies having problems latching on and feeding after birth, which may in turn have implications for bonding. However, the babies of women who've used opiates during labor don't appear to have greater problems putting on weight, which would be expected. And the claim that opiates put a baby at risk by depressing its respiratory system is considered by many to be exaggerated.

● More recent Swedish research links the extensive use of painkillers in labor to the increased likelihood of substance abuse later in life. Others suggest possible long-lasting effects on intellectual and behavioral development.

natural pain relief

Hypnosis

This can be an excellent way of treating physical pain as well as fear and anxiety (*see* page 103). The technique is to visualize yourself in a calm place to distract you from your discomfort. As you focus on breathing and serene thoughts, the uterus becomes less tense and opens up.

Massage

A lower back massage can alleviate some suffering, although not all women like being massaged once labor is under way.

Warm water

Standing in the shower letting warm water splash on your back can temporarily alleviate back pain. Alternatively, submerge your belly in warm water. The pressure underwater balances the pressure inside the uterus, providing relief. Deep tubs, known as birthing tubs, are available.

Heated packs

Applying warm compresses to your back is another way of soothing pain. Make one by filling a cotton sock with dry, uncooked rice and heating it in the microwave. You can stretch the sock into different positions on your body as it slowly releases heat.

Changing position

Leaning against a wall or walking around can ease some of the pressure. If you have back pain, get on your hands and knees. Combining changes of position with a rocking movement can help relieve pressure and tension.

Visualization

Imagining the birth process, from the first contractions to your final position for delivery and the emotion of the birth can help you feel more at home in this state when it actually happens. Imagine squatting, kneeling on all fours, or standing. Repeat a positive mantra as you picture each spasm. Proactive, positive meditation will help ease you into the real event.

Birthing balls

A birthing ball is the same as the large, soft, air-filled balls you see in fitness centers. Simply kneel and stretch your arms out over the ball, resting your head on top of it. Or sit on it and rock your pelvis backward and forward, which will also strengthen your back and abdominal muscles.

Soothing music and visual imagery

Listening to soothing music and looking at a wonderfully relaxing image can help distract you from discomfort.

Acupuncture

Acupuncture is safe to use throughout pregnancy. In the third trimester, acupuncture may encourage a head-down position for the baby, and during labor it is used to relieve pain, boost energy, and encourage contractions.

Acupressure

Acupressure can be used to reduce pain and relieve stress by stimulating the release of endorphins (natural painkillers). It involves pressing certain points on the body with fingers, knuckles, or palms, a technique you can learn yourself.

TENS

The purpose of a TENS machine (Transcutaneous Electrical Nerve Stimulation) is to trigger the release of endorphins. Electrodes are placed on your back and an electric current is passed through them: you control the amount of current. TENS machines will not harm mother or baby. I sometimes suggest using a TENS machine on acupressure points.

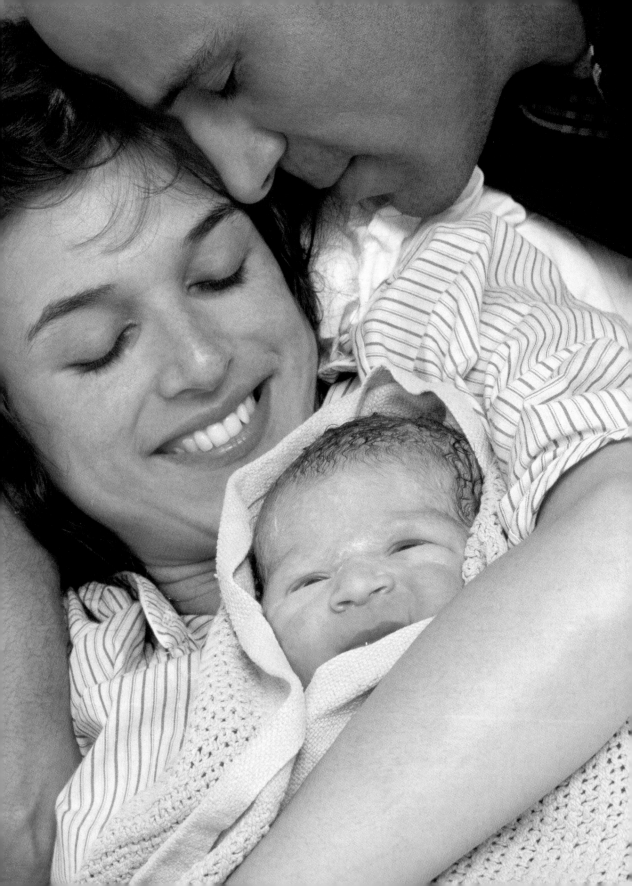

AFTER THE BIRTH

the first moments

The first moments following birth are truly amazing, no matter what type of delivery you've had. The joy I have witnessed as a midwife is boundless: feelings of relief that the birth is over and the baby is fine, followed by a sense of accomplishment and completeness, as well as exhaustion and euphoria.

MEETING YOUR BABY

Most hospitals now encourage immediate skin-to-skin contact between mother and baby, so your baby will be delivered onto your stomach. Babies usually breathe almost as soon as they're out of the birth canal, but in case your baby doesn't, there will be a pediatrician on hand who will clear his airways, administer a little oxygen, and kick start the breathing process. The first breath your baby takes is vitally important. He is now dependent on oxygen and his own ability to breathe.

From the minute he is born, your baby starts using his five senses to the full: looking at your face, smelling your smell, hearing your voice, being aware of your touch, tasting your skin, feeling your warmth. Imagine how cold it must be suddenly coming out into the world.

Your baby's brain starts to react to totally different stimuli from those it received in the uterus. He can see well and focus clearly on objects about 10in (25cm) away; he can tell the difference between shapes and patterns. Research suggests that newborns prefer stripes and angles to circular shapes, and yet faces are the most fascinating objects to your newborn baby. The epinephrine

After nine months of anticipation, finally meeting your new baby gives rise to feelings of euphoria and joy.

rush experienced during the birth takes some time to wear off, so your newborn is likely to be alert and will gaze back at you.

FOCUS ON BONDING

Bonding is sometimes described as a magical thing that is supposed to happen the instant you see your baby. This makes women panic if it doesn't happen right away. Some new mothers are in pain, or they're very uncomfortable or exhausted to the point that they cannot hold their baby, and they feel guilty as a result. If you have had a traumatic delivery and the baby is bruised, or maybe its head is a little misshapen, you may be shocked because your image of a beautiful baby being placed in your arms falls a little short of reality.

SEPARATION FROM YOUR BABY

Some babies need to go to the special care unit once they are born, either because they are very premature (*see* pages 114–15) or because they have a medical problem and need intensive treatment and monitoring. If your newborn goes to a unit, you will be taken to see him as soon as is practical and then encouraged to spend as much time as possible with him. Touching and stroking your baby will help you get to know each other and will help with the bonding process.

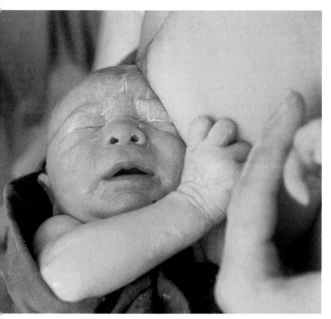

Early skin-to-skin contact is encouraged by most hospitals —your baby will probably be delivered onto your stomach.

Feel-good hormones usually kick in soon, but you may feel more of a sense of panic and need to sleep, or at least rest, before things start to improve.

Most mothers respond automatically the moment they see their baby looking vulnerable and in need of protection, and will instinctively reach out. Babies need to be loved, not just to satisfy an emotional need but as a biological necessity. They need the warmth and comfort of cuddles in order to flourish.

The maternal instinct is very strong, and your baby has ways of attaching you to him initially. He will lie in your arms, quietly looking up at you: his smell will appeal to you and vice versa. And the first feeding is an essential part of the bonding process—your baby will soon recognize the smell of your milk.

In these first few hours important connections are made in your baby's brain as he begins to become aware of warmth and comfort from others. These early experiences have a great impact on his mental well-being and later ability to process emotions.

FIRST HOURS AFTER BIRTH

The first few hours after the birth are different for every woman, and depend on the type of delivery experience. Some women sail through, feeling deliriously happy and on a high from which it will take a while to come down; others feel exhausted, anxious, and traumatized by delivery, and this can leave an impression that lasts for months.

It is important to get a couple of hours' sleep as soon as you can after the birth. Your baby needs emotional security, and for you to be emotionally present in the early days you need to rebuild your stores of energy. How you react to your baby and to the situations that arise will depend on how tired you are, so no matter how tempting it is to keep going while you are on a high, make sure you get the rest you need.

RECOVERING FROM A DIFFICULT BIRTH

I believe that the birth experience you have, whether or not you need a cesarean section or have a forceps or vacuum delivery, will be shaped by the support and expertise of those around you.

We are starting to see an increasing number of mothers who have experienced post-traumatic stress as the result of a negative birth experience— this can develop weeks or months after delivery, and can affect the bonding process. If you find you are suffering from this, go back and see your practitioner so that you can talk through the birth process, because this can help resolve the situation and improve how you feel.

Assisted deliveries

Babies who need to be delivered by forceps or vacuum often experience high levels of stress, and they may feel pain and be bruised at birth. These babies are often irritable and they tend to cry more and are harder to comfort, all of which affects the bonding process.

Often the mother is very sore and bruised as a result of the delivery, too. If you have had stitches, the skin surrounding them swells as the wound starts to heal and sitting down can be very uncomfortable. Sitting on a rubber ring or placing ice packs or local anesthetic cream on the perineum can help.

Birth by cesarean section

If you had a planned cesarean section using a spinal or an epidural anesthetic, you will have been awake and are likely to have had a happy experience. Such births happen very quickly, and mothers see their babies within minutes of going into the operating room. The whole procedure usually takes about an hour because the surgeon then has to carefully repair the uterus and the layers of tissue that were cut through to reach it.

On the other hand, if you had an emergency cesarean section, that became necessary because of a problem during labor, this sudden turn of events is likely to have been very stressful. You may be left with a feeling of disappointment or failure because you didn't give birth "naturally." It is important for you to remember that this emergency operation would not have been undertaken unless it was felt that your health or that of your baby was at serious risk. If the outcome is the safe delivery of a healthy baby then in no way should this be seen as any sort of failure.

Your physical recovery from a cesarean section may take some time, but it can be helped along tremendously with the right nutritional backup. For example, vitamins C and E are very important for wound healing, and zinc and selenium will boost your immunity and help protect against infection.

BONDING WITH YOUR PREMATURE BABY

Through positive touch (that is, touch that produces a positive reaction from the baby) and massage, you can play a role in helping your baby recover during its time in the NICU. Stroking can help her breathe more easily, and letting your baby hold your finger may help calm her. If your baby is very sick, however, touching might cause bruising or sleep disturbance. Always ask the nurses' advice.

Even though your baby is very tiny, you'll soon be able to recognize signs of whether to continue or to stop. She may arch her back or stretch her arms and legs to mean "stop"; if she is happy, her arms and legs will be relaxed, her facial expression will be soft, and her mouth may form an "O" shape.

As your baby grows and develops or her general health improves, you'll be able to touch her more and build up to cuddling. She may love being massaged and may sleep well and need less oxygen afterward. Once she is well enough and has grown enough for you to handle her with confidence, you can place her on your chest, tucked inside your clothing next to your skin. This is known as kangaroo care, and it warms and soothes the baby and will stimulate your milk production. Fathers and siblings can share close contact with the baby by doing this, too.

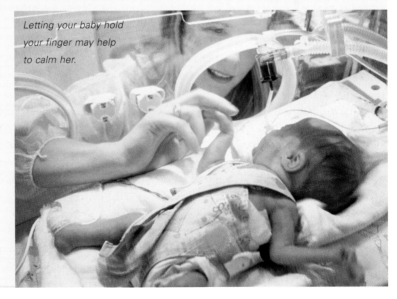

Letting your baby hold your finger may help to calm her.

life after birth

Trying to get new mothers to rest is difficult. I would love to return to the old midwifery practices, whereby mothers had a lying-in phase followed by a period of learning the ropes. New moms need guidance to give them confidence. These days, so many are just left to their own devices, and struggle as a result.

RECOVERING WELL

A new mother goes through a whole range of emotions in the first few days. In the hospital there is constant to-ing and fro-ing, bright lights and monitoring. Sleep deprivation is common: the day starts at 5:30am; there are no set visiting times; there is no routine. You're constantly waiting for the doctor's rounds; your turn in the shower; will you or won't you be discharged—it's very difficult. Others may barely see a hospital ward: you'll be sent home within hours of giving birth and expected to get on with it!

Most books paint a rosy picture of the early days of motherhood, spelling out what to do in the morning, the afternoon, and the evening. The reality is rather different. You do need a routine, so get up, feed your baby, have breakfast, shower—but then go back to bed and sleep, or at least rest. Wear an eye mask and pull the curtains around your bed to limit disturbance. Take time to really be with your baby. Forget about visitors coming, these early days should be spent doing nothing but sleeping, eating well, feeding, and resting in order to build up your reserves.

ARRIVING HOME

No one can prepare you for the first night at home. Even as a midwife who knew everything, on that first night it suddenly hit me that this little baby was my responsibility, 24 hours a day, seven days a

TIPS FOR NEW MOTHERS

- Stay in your nightclothes for as long as you can each day.
- Accept that the first night at home is probably going to be awful and your baby is going to be unsettled. I often find that sending the partner away and sleeping in another room that first night is very helpful. There is no point in you both being exhausted. You can then sleep in the following morning and your partner will be refreshed and can deal with the baby.
- Don't panic about not doing your housework—it doesn't matter.
- Forget about trying to get back into shape for at least six weeks.
- Don't travel long distances to visit relatives, and limit the number of visitors you have.
- Spend time as a couple getting to know your baby.

week, and there was no end to my shift. No matter how good your support is, the ultimate responsibility is with you. Sadly, with my second child, I suffered postpartum depression. I was up and around doing too much, cleaning, sleep deprived, not eating properly, and not building up my strength.

Spending the first few days focusing on getting to know your baby will pay dividends in the months ahead. Parents who are attuned to their babies' needs find they don't cry as easily and are more secure. Put your best effort into helping your baby sleep, bathing, changing, and feeding, and go with the flow. Don't impose hectic regimes or schedules. Slow down and learn how to deal with your baby. What you experience over the next few days and weeks represents a huge learning curve.

DEALING WITH STRESS

Having a baby is stressful. How well you cope with that stress will be reflected in your baby's experience. The more uninterrupted sleep you have, the more focused you are, the better you will cope. Focus on your family unit, and make sure you don't get side-tracked by small things. The stress control mechanisms you practiced during pregnancy will be just as useful now.

Like many new mothers, you may worry about how good you'll be at interpreting your baby's needs. But it's hard to get it wrong for a baby if you answer his basic needs for warmth, love, food, and to be changed into clean diapers. If you're anxious, you will have greater difficulty managing those needs, but in time you will build up confidence. Babies are creatures of habit: they like a regular pattern of events. You may not get anything else done but just accepting this fact will help you. Establishing a sleeping and feeding routine will not only keep the baby happy, it will keep you sane.

Use relaxation techniques to build up your reserves of energy and keep you calm. If you are tired and stressed you will be less able to manage a difficult baby, with the knock-on effect that your baby will seem more and more difficult. This becomes obvious when a mother who cannot settle her baby hands it to granny and the baby senses calm and stops crying immediately.

The way we respond to stress is one aspect of our emotional makeup. It is linked to the release of hormones and the behavior of neurotransmitters (chemical "messengers" used by nerve cells to communicate with each other). Our stress response was influenced in the first instance by how our parents handled our cries and demands when we were babies.

PART OF THE FAMILY

If you already have a child it is important to keep as much continuity as possible at home. It is perfectly normal for the arrival of a new family member to cause feelings of jealousy in siblings, possibly resulting in more clingy, naughty, or attention-seeking behavior in the early weeks. Make sure you give your first child plenty of cuddles and try to dedicate a little time every day to doing something together without the baby there—your partner or other family members can look after the baby for a while. Once your first child is confident that he still has your love and attention, he will begin to enjoy his new sibling.

You and your partner will quickly learn to interpret and respond to your baby's needs.

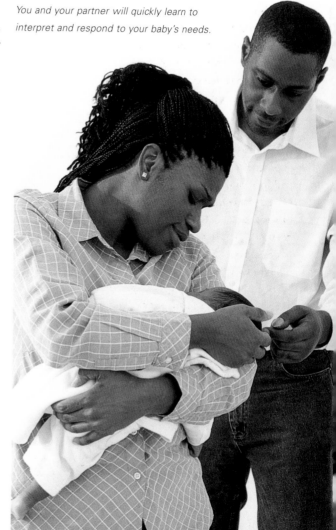

postpartum nutrition

Very often a women nurtures and looks after herself during pregnancy, but the focus quickly shifts after the birth from her needs to those of her baby. However, looking after your own nutrition during the postpartum period is vitally important for speeding up the healing process and for breastfeeding.

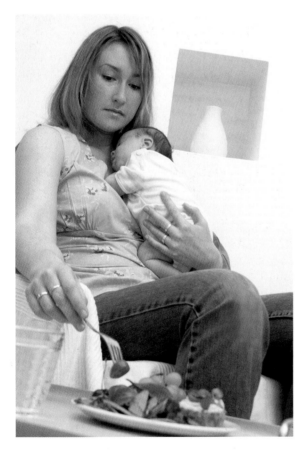

"you need to replenish nutrients after birth"

THE BREASTFEEDING CONNECTION

I understand absolutely that not every woman can or wants to breastfeed, but there is no better way of continuing the physical connection between you and your baby. She may be breathing on her own, but she is still reliant on you for food—through the breast rather than the placenta.

Oxytocin is the hormone that "powers" breastfeeding. This is also the hormone that causes your uterus to contract in labor, so it will help you get your figure back! It's known as the love or cuddle hormone because it stimulates warm, tender feelings toward your baby—and toward your partner, too! If you're emotionally stressed, the hormone will be blocked and will not allow you to let down milk successfully for breastfeeding. So, the relaxation techniques you used before and during labor will come in handy now, too.

The let-down process

Milk production is driven by the sucking action of your baby (*see* facing page). When your baby latches onto your breast and sucks, nerve endings in your nipple send messages to a part of your brain called the hypothalamus. This in turn instructs the pituitary gland to release two hormones: prolactin, which stimulates the breasts to start making milk; and oxytocin, which triggers the release of milk from your breasts for that feed.

KEY POSTPARTUM NUTRIENTS

The quality of your breast milk is affected by what you eat and how tired and stressed you are. If your body is not functioning smoothly, then your breast milk will not be at its best. Just as you did before your baby was born, you have to eat as healthily as you can in order to provide the raw materials for high-quality breast milk. It is recommended that you eat an extra 500 calories a day when breastfeeding. I would also recommend that you continue to take a multivitamin and mineral supplement to rebuild your stores of vital vitamins and minerals, which will have been depleted during the birth.

Pay particular attention to these nutrients:
• **Protein** The baby is now growing faster than ever and you should eat plenty of protein. You may even need to double the average two servings a day, or at least have one extra.
• **Calcium** Growing bones need plenty of calcium and milk is a rich source. If your intake does not provide enough for your baby's requirements, the mineral will be taken from your bones.
• **Iron** You have to replace blood lost during labor as well as make sure that your baby builds up sufficient reserves of iron. This mineral also helps with healing, protects against infection, and helps all the cells in your baby's body get enough oxygen to fuel growth.
• **Zinc** If your diet is deficient in zinc—and large amounts go to the baby and the placenta before birth—your breast milk will be too, and this mineral is vital for your baby's neurological development. Zinc is also important for your hormone production and healing. Depression is a common side effect of zinc deficiency.
• **Vitamin C** This is important for collagen production, which is part of the healing process, and for breastfeeding.

You also need to replenish silica, important if you suffer hair loss after pregnancy; B vitamins, particularly B_6; magnesium; and vitamin K (for the baby to store).

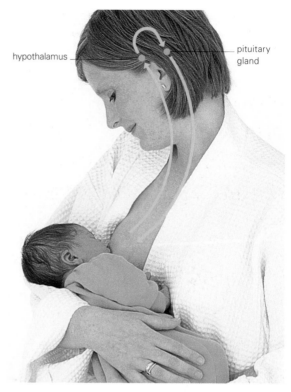

hypothalamus — pituitary gland

Your baby's sucking triggers the release of hormones in your brain, which tell your body to produce and release milk.

Eating well

It is a good idea to spread your food intake over five meals during the day: breakfast, lunch, afternoon snack, dinner, and evening snack. Since your body is continually producing milk you need to supply it with food at regular intervals.

You should also increase your water intake while breastfeeding. You may find that you are thirstier anyway, especially during a feeding, because part of the water you drink goes directly into the process of milk production.

THE EVER-IMPORTANT DHA

During her first year, your baby's brain will almost triple in weight to about 2lb 4oz (1kg). She requires essential fats to make cell membranes and to build up the protective coating around nerve fibers. Many of these fats come from your milk, which is why it is so important for you to keep up your intakes of fatty acids. Research also shows that if a mother has a good supply of DHA, she is less likely to suffer postpartum depression.

The DHA content in your diet is reflected in the amount of DHA passed on to the baby because she can't make her own until she is four to six months old. Infants who are breastfed have significantly greater amounts of DHA in their

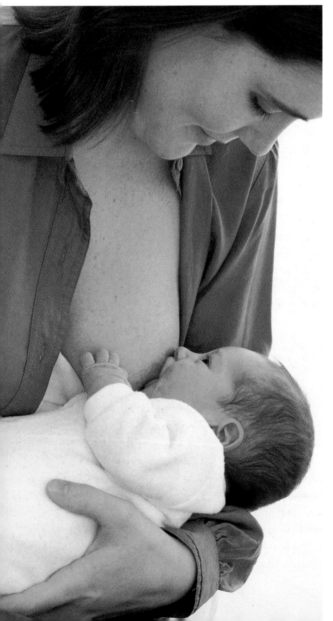

brains than those fed standard, nonenriched formula, although many formulas do now contain essential fatty acids.

DHA levels of premature infants are especially low since they miss much of the last trimester. In addition, premature babies are more likely to be bottle-fed formula because the sucking reflex isn't fully developed and they will use up valuable calories trying to suck from the breast. It can also take longer for the mother's milk to come in if the baby is born early. The majority of mothers express milk to feed to their babies until they are able to breastfeed.

THE BENEFITS OF BREAST MILK

The carbohydrates and fats in breast milk provide energy for your newborn to grow—fats are particularly important for brain development. In addition, breast milk contains a complete spectrum of proteins, ensuring your baby has all the necessary "building blocks" for generating new tissue, as well as all the valuable vitamins and minerals your baby needs.

Breast milk also includes antibodies that strengthen your baby's immune system. These antibodies represent a record of the diseases you have been exposed to and successfully fought off. Antibodies are especially important in colostrum, a thick, rich fluid that precedes milk. They give your newborn the edge in the survival stakes when she emerges from a sterile environment in which she had no exposure to germs. Antibodies help fight off germs and line the baby's gut, aiding digestion as well as immunity.

When our digestive tracts are working well, they contain huge numbers of beneficial bacteria to assist digestion. An infant's digestive tract needs these, too. I encourage all women, even those who are sure for whatever reason that they don't want to breastfeed, to do it for at least two to three

Your breast milk is designed exclusively to fulfill the needs of your baby, gving him the best possible start in life.

days. This way they will at least give their babies colostrum, which will pay enormous dividends in terms of their future health.

Arguments in favor of breastfeeding

• Breastfed babies are brainier. Recent studies indicate that they have an IQ 6–10 points higher than formula-fed babies, probably due to higher levels of essential fatty acids.
• Fat-soluble vitamins, such as vitamin D, in breast milk are absorbed more easily.
• Breast-fed babies are less likely to be obese.
• Breastfeeding helps you lose weight: the baby consumes about 500 calories a day.

WATCHING WHAT YOU EAT

You can eat most things while breastfeeding, but occasionally some foods may cause problems.
• Vegetables such as cabbage, onion, garlic, broccoli, brussels sprouts, cauliflower, peppers, cucumbers, and turnips can cause gas, so it's best not to eat too much of them until your baby's digestive system is better able to cope.
• Cow's milk products may cause symptoms of allergy in your baby such as diarrhea, runny nose, cough, or rash. Leave dairy products out of your diet for a couple of weeks, then reintroduce them, one at a time, and see if symptoms recur.

• Citrus fruits may produce the same allergic reaction. Do as above.
• Other potential allergens include eggs, wheat, corn, fish, nuts, and soy.
• Some herbs are toxic. Mint, sage, and parsley may dry up the milk supply; feverfew may increase the baby's heart rate; and St. John's wort, which is used to treat depression, may affect milk production. Use herbal teas with care unless you know what ingredients they contain. Fenugreek and fennel have traditionally been claimed to boost milk supply.
• Alcohol passes through to your milk, albeit in smaller quantities—30–90 minutes after you've drunk it. If you want to have more than a couple of glasses of wine a week, drink after the last feeding of the day.
• Caffeine may make your baby fractious and interfere with her sleep. She can't get rid of it easily so if your intakes are high it builds up in her body.
• Nicotine is not easily absorbed by a baby and is quickly metabolized but, if you smoke heavily (more than 20 cigarettes a day), milk production may be reduced and the baby may suffer symptoms such as vomiting, diarrhea, increased heart rate, and restlessness, as well as being more prone to colic and respiratory ailments such as asthma. Don't smoke near your baby, and try to give up.

LOSING WEIGHT FOLLOWING THE BIRTH

A woman builds up her fat reserves by the end of pregnancy in order to see her through the early breastfeeding period. It is important not to try to lose weight quickly after the birth while you are breastfeeding or the quality and quantity of your milk will be reduced.

Fat accounts for 60 percent of the calories provided in breast milk, and your body stores are essential to give your baby good quality milk in the quantities he needs. You may find that some weight falls off naturally while you're breastfeeding, especially as the baby grows faster and gets hungrier.

After the birth, you are healing and your baby is developing, especially his brain, respiratory system, and pancreas. A baby is born with only about half the number of alveoli (air sacs) in his lungs that he will eventually need, and lung development continues for two years.

If that development is impaired due to inadequate nutrition or infection, the lungs will not reach their full size or function properly.

So, if you must lose weight, leave it until breastfeeding is well established, at least three months after the birth, and preferably after your baby is weaned. And take it off slowly: it took you nine months to put the weight on, so try to take it off just as gradually.

caring for your baby

Most of us respond to our babies automatically. We understand their signals and react to their fundamental needs. By communicating with your baby, even on this basic level, you are helping his nervous system mature. His early experiences of human interaction mold his emotional development.

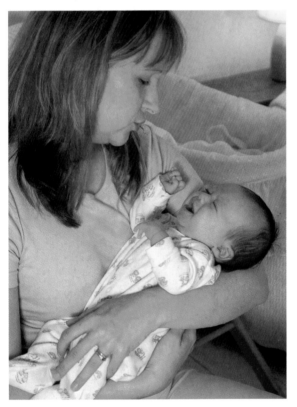

"remember that crying babies do not mean bad mothers"

WHAT TO EXPECT OF YOUR BABY

Newborn babies sleep for between 16 and 20 hours a day. The fact that most babies spend much of their time asleep gives you a chance to recover from the birth and get used to your new life. Make sure you don't spend all their sleep time cleaning, tidying up, washing, or shopping—even spending just half an hour lying on your bed, relaxing or meditating, will help you cope.

It might take your baby as long as six weeks to distinguish between night and day, and from then on he will be awake more during the day than at night. Some babies find it more difficult to establish a night-and-day sleep pattern than others. This may be because their brains are maturing more slowly, or, if they're growing fast, they may be unable to go through the night without having something to eat.

Between about four weeks and three months old, babies tend to become more alert. They can move their heads and will become fascinated by their surroundings. They'll have two or three naps during the day lasting for a couple of hours, and they'll probably sleep for about eight hours at night. From four to six months babies are more active and mobile. They might have two naps of two to three hours each, and then, if you are lucky, they'll sleep for 10–12 hours a night as well. Not all babies will follow this pattern, but it gives you the general idea.

At night time, a regular, gentle wind-down from the day is very important. Feeding, cuddling, rocking, and soft music all help. Very small babies need to be almost asleep before being put down: most young babies like to go to sleep in their parents' arms. Make sure your baby is at the right temperature (97.7–98.6°F/36.5–37°C).

CRYING

Considering how small they are, most babies can cry quite loudly. Their parents are programmed to react to this stimulus, of course: they become concerned and, if a baby cries a lot, anxious.

When a baby cries, it can mean "I'm hungry," "My diaper needs changing," "I'm tired," or uncomfortable in some other way. You will come to understand the difference as the weeks go by. There are many books on how to get your baby into a routine, and that's fine. But your baby is an individual and you are an individual and you both need to find the way for yourselves, together. By all means use books as guides, but you don't have to follow them to the letter.

As a parent, you must take the lead. You know better than your baby does. Remember that the responses he develops will up to a point reflect your response, so always think through what you are doing. Also remember that crying babies do not mean bad mothers. Don't take your baby's crying personally: you're doing your best to interpret your baby's needs.

YOUR EMOTIONS

You will run the whole gamut of emotions in the days and weeks to come. You will get cross and frustrated, which is perfectly normal. You may also feel your confidence slipping away. The best way to build this back up is to spend time with your baby.

It's easy to see why these emotional surges happen. Immediately after the birth, you're elated; then your milk comes in and your breasts might be sore, and your baby may be irritable because he can't suck easily. Your hormones are all over the place and you crash down emotionally. The hormones estrogen and progesterone drop dramatically within hours of delivery, and so do the endorphins that helped you cope with pain and made you joyful.

Not everyone experiences this, but almost all women feel lesser or greater degrees of fatigue, discomfort, and emotional roller-coasting in the early days and weeks after the birth—one minute you're laughing, the next you're sobbing your heart out. Try to get out to meet other new mothers, from your prenatal class for example, or join a postpartum exercise or yoga class. Accept any offers of help from family and friends, and if things really do start to get you down, wrap your baby up and take him out for a walk. You will always come back feeling happier.

COPING WITH CRYING

- All babies cry when they're hungry. If you think your baby has had enough food, but he doesn't agree, then letting him suck your finger or a pacifier may be a suitable substitute.
- Most babies like a regular rhythm of feeding and sleeping. Try to maintain their routine so they don't become unsettled.
- Babies like to be rocked because this happened to them all the time when they were in the uterus. Rock your baby in your arms, in his carriage, or sitting in a rocking chair.
- Carry your baby in a sling, keeping him close to you.
- Check to see if your baby might be too hot or too cold.
- Change your baby's diaper. Some babies are sensitive to discomfort.
- Your baby might be in need of stimulation, or be feeling abandoned if he is on his own and in need of a cuddle. On the other hand, over-stimulation might make your baby irritable.
- Playing music can be soothing, as can chatting, singing a lullaby, and reading to your baby (it's never too soon to start story-telling). Rhythmic noise and vibration, from a vacuum cleaner or washing machine for example, can also help.

stimulating your baby

Once outside the uterus, your baby continues to develop at an astonishing rate. Each time she is stimulated—through sound, touch, taste, sight, smell, and intellectual and emotional interactions—thousands of new connections are made in the brain. The more she is stimulated, the more she will learn.

NURTURING NATURE

Once in the outside world, the stimuli your baby's brain receives are much more numerous—it is constantly receiving, assimilating, and sorting information. Most stimulation comes through your baby's interactions with adults. As you talk to your baby, smile at her, and cuddle her, she begins to associate these interactions with comfort and pleasure. The foundations of her emotional and physical health and well-being are being laid down. Being stimulated and nurtured in this way is the best encouragement to development.

The first year of life is very important for further brain development, which requires nourishment and stimulation. An enriched environment boosts the number of synapses (connections) made by each neuron by as much as 25 percent (*see* pages 92–3). In a neglected, understimulated child, the establishment of new synapses and the destruction of under-used neurons becomes unbalanced.

Research indicates that children who are not played with and who are rarely touched or stimulated, develop a brain up to 30 percent smaller than would be expected for their stage of development. Just as in the uterus there were "windows of opportunity" for the fetus' crucial development, there are a number of critical times for an infant to learn new skills. Once these periods are past, particular areas of the brain will have

STIMULATING YOUR BABY'S SENSES

Your baby wants to be with you: spend as much time together as possible. Remember, in the grand scheme of things, your baby's early months are a very short time indeed.

- Cuddle and gently rock your baby. Babies love to be rocked because it reminds them of being in the uterus.
- Talk to your baby: she will recognize your voice from the outset and will find it soothing.

- Play music and sing to your baby.
- Babies seem to like mobiles consisting of contrasting black and white patterns.
- Introduce your baby to colors and slightly more complex patterns from 6–8 weeks onward.
- Show your baby her reflection in the mirror.
- Give your baby different textures to feel as she develops.

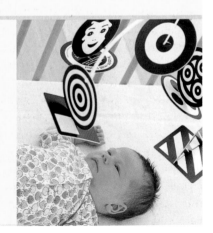

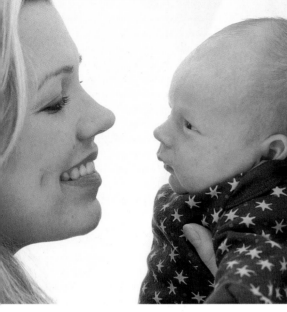

Talking to and touching your baby will have an enormous impact on her emotional and intellectual development.

BABY MASSAGE

Touch is so important. By three months old, the part of your baby's brain involved in detecting touch is more active. Babies that are massaged regularly are more alert and active when they're awake; they fall asleep better, and gain more weight. They also tend to have a better temperament, be more sociable, and are less likely to cry.

The more you appreciate the importance of touch, the greater sense it seems to make to massage your baby. There are many benefits: massage can help your baby's circulatory, respiratory, and digestive systems, and encourage growth. It is also good for stimulating muscles. You can teach yourself massage using books and videos or through organizations that offer classes.

There is a difference of opinion among professionals about when you should start massaging your baby. Some believe between three and four months, but I think you can start right away as long as your baby is healthy and you choose a time when he is alert and ready for some stimulation. Don't massage just before a feeding or too soon after. Make sure you've got lots of time and concentrate on what you're doing—don't, for example, try to massage while you watch television. And don't break the spell by making sudden movements.

You need baby massage oil, a warm room, and a comfortable space for your baby. Make sure she is not cold, turn the lights down, and wash and warm your hands before you begin.

become less able to make new connections, so the skills they are associated with are less easily learned. The right input at the right time is what is required. But intensive "hot-housing" is not the answer either.

EMOTIONAL DEVELOPMENT

During the first couple of months of life, your baby's emotions are fairly uncomplicated: she is either content or upset. But then the "circuitry" for emotional development starts to be laid down in the brain, and is mostly in place by the time she reaches the age of 10. Your child will gradually develop a more sophisticated range of emotions along with her sense of being an individual. Happiness and contentment result from a loving, caring environment.

During the first year it is especially important to be in tune emotionally with your baby as this is a critical window of development and your baby will mirror your responses. Developing an understanding of what makes your baby anxious or upset, happy or excited will help you manage the inevitable highs and lows of this stage in your baby's life.

TALKING

Research shows that babies and infants who are consistently talked to from an early age have significantly higher IQ scores than those whose parents are less communicative. If babies are not touched and held a lot during the first six months of their lives, they are more likely to become apathetic and neurotic. When I was nursing, sometimes babies came into the unit who were described as "failure to thrive" babies. Often, when we observed their parents we could see that the babies weren't talked to or held very often.

nutrient sources

Much of the advice in this book relies on nutrients that are key to a healthy pregnancy. In this quick reference guide you will find the best food sources for all the important food groups, vitamins, and minerals described throughout the book.

PROTEIN
chicken
roast beef
sirloin steak
bolognaise sauce
tuna
cod
cheddar cheese
cottage cheese
baked beans
kidney beans
eggs
milk
canned corn
hummus
almonds
Brazil nuts
cashew nuts
walnuts
pine nuts
oatmeal (raw or cooked)
frozen peas
baked or mashed potato
seedless raisins

brown rice
pumpkin seeds
sunflower seeds
soy milk
lentils
cooked spinach
wholewheat spaghetti
canned tomatoes
tofu
quorn
wholemeal bread
plain yogurt

Glycine (amino acid)
cod
tuna
chicken
beef
eggs
milk
kidney beans
baked beans
black-eyed peas
lentils

CARBOHYDRATE
Complex carbohydrates
wholewheat pasta
spaghetti
brown rice
sweet potatoes
wholemeal breads
granary, brown, and pita breads
wholegrain cereals
oats
muesli
corn
oatcakes
legumes

Simple carbohydrates
fruit
refined white flour
processed food

ESSENTIAL FATTY ACIDS
DHA (an omega-3 EFA)
seafood
coldwater fish, including organic

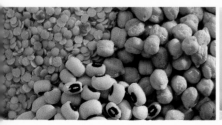
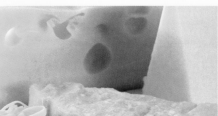
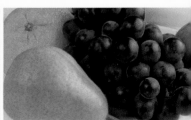

or wild salmon, sardines, tuna, herring, mackerel and cod
seaweed
eggs
walnuts
pumpkin seeds
flaxseeds and flaxseed oil
hempseeds and hempseed oil
Brazil nuts
sesame seeds
avocados
dark, leafy green vegetables such as kale, spinach, mustard greens and collards

Arachidonic acid (an omega-6 EFA)
flaxseeds and flaxseed oil
hempseeds and hempseed oil
grapeseed oil
pumpkin seeds
pine nuts
sunflower seeds
olives
olive oil

MINERALS
Calcium
milk and other dairy products
spinach
broccoli
parsley
watercress
canned fish with edible bones such as sardines and tuna

shellfish
oranges
pinto beans
lettuce greens
parsley
watercress
cottage cheese
hard cheese
kelp
flaxseeds
tofu
figs
sesame seeds

Iron
meat (lean)
fish
chicken
eggs
kelp
molasses
pumpkin seeds
broccoli
oatmeal
spinach
parsley
dried apricots/figs
prunes
enriched grain products

Zinc
meat (lean)
fish
chicken
seafood

eggs
pumpkin seeds
sunflower seeds
whole grains
ginger root
split peas
rye
oats
parsley
mushrooms
brewer's yeast
wheatgerm

Magnesium
almonds
green leafy vegetables
tofu
pulses
rye
molasses
brown rice
bananas
dried apricots/figs
barley

Manganese
pecans
spinach
Brazil nuts
barley
oats
rye
raisins
brown rice
green leafy vegetables

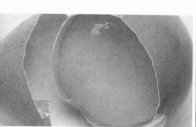

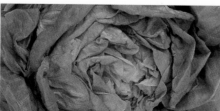

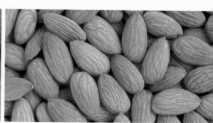

carrots
Brussels sprouts
ginger
eggs
parsley
thyme
walnuts

Phosphorus
fish
poultry
meat
eggs
legumes
milk and milk products
nuts
wholegrain cereals

Potassium
bananas
apples
pineapple
dried apricots
peaches
melons
avocados
carrots
tomatoes
leafy green vegetables
potatoes
asparagus
lean meats
whole grains
legumes
sunflower seeds

Selenium
tuna and herring
Brazil nuts
wheatgerm oil
oats
barley
orange juice
turnips
garlic
butter
brown rice
wheatgerm and bran

Iodine
fish
seaweed
iodized salt

Choline
beef
fish
egg yolks
iceberg lettuce
peanuts

VITAMINS
Vitamin A
whole milk
butter
eggs
fruit and vegetables containing
carotenes (carrots, sweet potatoes,
peppers, tomatoes, spinach,
sweetcorn, squash, apricots, pink
grapefruit, watermelon)

Folic acid
blackeye peas
beans and pulses
lentils
green leafy vegetables
asparagus
oatmeal
dried figs
avocados
egg yolk
yeast extract
milk and milk products

Vitamin B$_6$
wholegrains
chickpeas
seeds
raisins
lentils
bananas
avocados
cabbage
molasses
milk products
eggs

Vitamin B$_{12}$
sardines
trout
salmon
lamb
eggs
lean beef
Edam cheese
cottage cheese

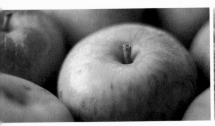
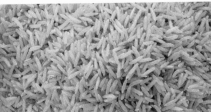
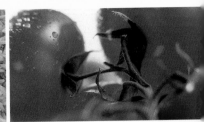

Vitamin C

oranges and juice
melon
mango
lemon
kiwi fruit
blackcurrants
papaya
green and red peppers
tomatoes
parsley
watercress
broccoli
spinach
cauliflower

Vitamin D

canned salmon and tuna
egg yolks
dark green leafy vegetables
sunlight on the skin

Vitamin E

wholegrains
nuts
seeds
organic cold-pressed nut and
seed oils (sesame, walnut)

Vitamin K

green leafy vegetables
egg yolks
safflower oil
molasses
cauliflower

HIGH AND LOW GI FOODS

The glycaemic index operates on a scale of 1–100 and is based on how quickly a food is digested, metabolized and released into the blood as glucose (*see* page 61). Foods with a lower GI ranking make us feel fuller for longer and encourage stable blood sugar.

Low GI foods—that is, 40 and below on the index. Eat as many of these slow-release foods as possible.
● Apples, plums, pears, dried apricots, peaches, cherries
● All legumes—lentils, kidney beans, haricot beans (baked beans), cannellini beans, butter beans, chickpeas
● Green leafy vegetables—broccoli, Brussels sprouts, cauliflower, cabbage, snow peas, leeks, green beans, onions, avocados, zucchini, peppers
● Wholegrain cereals, wholegrain rye bread, barley, yogurt, nuts

Medium GI foods—41–60 on the index. Include moderate amounts of these in your diet.
● Grapes, under-ripe bananas, mango, figs, kiwi fruit
● Corn, peas, raw carrots, beetroot, boiled and sweet potatoes
● Oatcakes, noodles, popcorn, wholewheat pasta, wholemeal bread, brown basmati rice

High GI foods—above 60 on the index. Eat these foods in moderation, with protein or fat. Avoid completely refined and processed foods with added sugars and sweeteners.
● Baked and mashed potatoes, cooked carrots, parsnip, swede, winter squash
● Ripe bananas, watermelon, raisins
● White bread, white rice and pasta, couscous, sugared breakfast cereals
● Sugar, jam, honey, sweets

ANTIOXIDANTS

prunes
blueberries
blackberries
strawberries
red grapes
plums
garlic
kale
brussels sprouts
alfalfa sprouts
broccoli
cauliflower
red pepper
green pepper
kidney beans
tomatoes
spinach

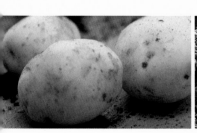
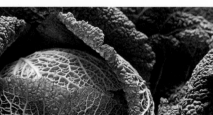
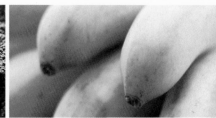

resources & references

BACKGROUND READING

Barker DJB. *The Best Start in Life*. Century; 2003.

Barker DJP. The developmental origins of chronic adult disease. *Acta Paediatrica*. 2004;446(suppl): 26–33.

Barker DJP. *The Developmental Origins of Well-being*. The Royal Society; August 11, 2004, online.

Barker DJP. *Mothers, Babies and Health in Later Life*. Churchill Livingstone; 1998.

Bensadoun P, Nathanielsz PW. *Life Before Birth: The Challenges of Fetal Development*. WH Freeman; 1996

Dye FJ. *Human Life Before Birth*. Harwood Academic Publishers; 2000.

Gluckman P, Hanson M. *The Fetal Matrix: Evolution, Development and Disease*. Cambridge University Press; 2005.

Moore KL, Persaud TVN. *Before We Are Born: Essentials of Embryology and Birth Defects*. Saunders; 2003.

Odent M. *Primal Health: Understanding the Critical Period between Conception and the First Birthday*. Clairview Books; 2002.

Verny T, MD with Kelly J. *The Secret Life Of the Unborn Child: How You Can Prepare Your Baby for a Happy, Healthy Life*. Dell; 1982.

FERTILITY

Abell A, Ernst E, Bonde JP.High sperm density among members of organic farmers' association. *Lancet*. 1994;343:1498.

Bianco A et al. Pregnancy outcome at age 40 and older. *Obstetrics and Gynecology* 1996;87:917–22.

Carlson E et el. Evidence for decreasing quality of semen during past 50 years. BMJ. 1992;305(6854):609–13.

Gilbert WM et al. Childbearing beyond age 40: pregnancy outcome in 24,032 cases. *Obstetrics and Gynecology* 1999;93:9–14.

Goverde HJM, Dekker HS, Janssen HJG et al. Semen quality and frequency of smoking and alcohol consumption—an explorative study. *International Journal of Fertility* 1995;40:135–8.

Kreset DM. Declining sperm counts. *British Medical Journal* 1996;312:457–8.

CONCEPTION AND PREGNANCY

Burton GJ, Jauniaux E. Placental oxidative stress; from miscarriage to preeclampsia. *Journal of Society for Gynecological Investigation*. 2004; 11:342–352.

Hempstock J, Jauniaux E, Greenwold N, Burton GJ. The contribution of placental oxidative stress to early pregnancy failure. *Human Pathology*. 2003;34:1265–1275.

Kitzinger S. *The New Pregnancy and Childbirth*, Penguin; 1997.

Nilsson L and Hamberger L. *A Child Is Born*. Delta Trade Paperbacks; 2004

Page K. *The Physiology of the Human Placenta*. UCL Press; 1993.

Regan L. *I'm Pregnant!* DK Publishing, Inc; 2005.

Wesson N. *Home Birth: Comprehensive Guide to Planning Childbirth at Home*, Vermilion; 1996.

Wesson N. *Labour Pain*. Vermilion; 1999.

NUTRITION

Barker DJP. Fetal origins of coronary heart disease. *British Medical Journal* 1995;311:171–4.

Barker DJP, Osmond C. Infant mortality, childhood nutrition, and ischaemic heart disease in England and Wales. Barker DJP, Osmond C, Winter PD, Margetts BM, Simmonds SJ. Weight in infancy and death from ischaemic heart disease. *Lancet*. 1989;2:577–580.

Bothwell TH. *Iron requirements in pregnancy and strategies to meet them*. [Review] [64 refs] *American Journal of Clinical Nutrition* 2000;72(suppl): 257S–264S.

Campbell DM, Hall MH, Barker DJP, Cross J, Shiell AW and Godfrey KM. Diet in pregnancy and the offspring's blood pressure 40 years later. *British Journal of Obstetrics and Gynaecology*. 1996;103:273–280.

Eriksson JG, Forsén T, Tuomilehto J, Jaddoe VWV, Osmond C, Barker, DJP. Effects of size at birth and childhood growth on the insulin resistance syndrome in elderly individuals. *Diabetologia*. 2002;45:342–348.

Godfrey K, Robinson S, Barker DJP. Osmond C, Cox V. Maternal nutrition in early and late pregnancy in relation to placental and fetal growth. *British Medical Journal*. 1996;312:410–414. *Lancet*. 1986; i:1077–81.

Hytten FE. Nutrition. *Clinical Physiology in Obstetrics*, Hytten FE, Chamberlain G (Eds). Blackwell Scientific Publications; 1980.

Institute of Medicine. *Nutrition During Pregnancy: Part I Weight Gain, Part II: Nutrient Supplements*. National Academy Press (Washington DC); 1990.

Morgan JB, Dickerson JWT. *Nutrition in Early Life*. Wiley; 2002.

UK Dept. of Health. *Dietary Reference Values for Food Energy and Nutrients for the United Kingdom*. HMSO 1991.

Vollset SE et al. Plasma total homocysteine, pregnancy complications, and adverse pregnancy outcomes: the Hordaland homocysteine study. *American Journal of Clinical Nutrition* 2000;71:962–8.

ENVIRONMENT

Colburn T, Dumanoski D, Myers JP. *Our Stolen Future: Are We Threatening our Fertility, Intelligence, and Survival?* Plume Books; 1997.

Hruska KS, Furth PA, Seifer DB, et al.

Environmental factors in infertility. *Clinical Obstetrics and Gynecology* 2000;43:821–9 Schettler T et al. *Generations at Risk: Reproductive Health and the Environment.* MIT Press; 2000.

LIFESTYLE

Abel EL. Infertility increases when alcohol and marijuana combined. *Teratology.* 1985;31:35–40.

Bolumar F, Olsen J, Boldsen J, and the European Study Group on Infertility and Subfecundity. Smoking reduces fecundity: a European multicenter study on infertility and subfecundity. *American Journal of Epidemiology* 1996;143: 578–87.

Grodstein F, Goldman MB, Cramer DW. Infertility in women and moderate alcohol use. *American Journal of Public Health.* 1994;84:1429–52.

Yazigi, R. Cocaine and abnormal offspring. *Journal of the American Medical Association* October 1991;66(14).

FETAL DEVELOPMENT

Chamberlain DB. Is there intelligence before birth? *Pre- and Perinatal Psychology Journal* 1992;6(3):217–237.

Hepper PG. Foetal "soap" addiction. *Lancet.* June 1988;11:1347–8.

Hepper PG. An examination of fetal learning before and after birth. *Irish Journal of Psychology* 1991;12:95–107.

Hepper PG, Scott D, Shahdullah S. Newborn and fetal response to maternal voice. *Journal of Reproductive and Infant Psychology* 1993;11:147–53.

Lalande NM, Hetu R, Lambert J. Is occupational noise exposure during pregnancy a risk factor of damage to the auditory system of the fetus? *American Journal of Independent Medicine* 1986;10:427–435.

Montagu A. *Touching: The Human Significance of the Skin,* Harper Paperbacks; 1986.

Olsen J, Rachootin P, Schiodt A et al. Tobacco use, alcohol consumption, and infertility, *International Journal of*

*Epidemiol*ogy 1983;12:179–184.

Pasamanick B. Pregnancy experience and the development of behavior disorders in children. *American Journal of Psychiatry.* 1956; 112:613–617.

Rovee-Collier CK, Lipsitt LP. *Learning, adaptation, and memory in the newborn,* in Stratton, P.M. (Ed) *Psychobiology of the human newborn.* Wiley & Sons; 1982:147–190.

Smith E, Hammonds-Ehlers M, Clark M et al. Occupational exposures and risk of female infertility. *Journal of Occupational and Environmental Medicine* 1997;39:138–147.

de Vries JIP, Visser GHA, Prectl FR II. The emergence of fetal behaviour II. quantitative aspects. *Early Human Development* 1985;12:99–120.

NURTURING

Adamson-Macedo EN, Attree JLA. *The importance of systematic stroking, TAC-TIC therapy, British Journal of Midwifery* 1994;2(6): 264–269.

Chamberlain DB. The cognitive newborn: a scientific update. *British Journal of Psychotherapy* 1987;4(1): 30–71.

Chamberlain DB. *The sentient prenate: What every parent should know, Pre- and Perinatal Psychology Journal* 1994; 1:9–31.

DeCasper A, Fifer W. Of human bonding: newborns prefer their mother's voice.*Science.* 1980;208:1174–1176.

Gerhardt S. *Why Love Matters: How Affection Shapes a Baby's Brain.* Brunner-Routledge; 2004.

Verny T, Weintraub P. *Nurturing the Unborn Child.* Olmstead Press; 2000.

USEFUL WEBSITES

Zita West Clinic
www.zitawest.com for information on the Zita West Better Baby Program

American Association for Premature Infants
www.raapi-online.org

American College of Nurse Midwives
www.midwife.org

American College of Obsetricians and Gynecologists
www.acog.org

American Osteopathic Association
www.osteopathic.org

Association for Children with Down Syndrome
www.acds.org

Birth Defect Research for Children
www.birthdefects.org

Ferre Institute, Inc. (advice on infertility)
www.ferre.org

Healthy Mothers, Healthy Babies Coalition
www.hmhb.org

Hydrocephalus Association
www.hydroass.org

International Childbirth Education Association
www.icea.org

National Center for Education and Maternal and Child Health
www.ncemch.org

International Cesarean Awareness Network
www.ican-online.org

Mommies Enduring Neonatal Disease (MEND)
www.mend.org

Mothers of Supertwins
www.mostonline.org

Postpartum Assistance for Mothers
www.postpartumassistance.com

Preeclampsia Foundation
www.preeclampsi.org

Resolve, Inc. (advice on infertility)
www.resolve.org

The Smile Train (international charity for children born with a cleft palate)
www.smiletrain.org

index

acknowledgments

Zita West would like to thank Jude Garlick for helping her collate the material for this book and write it. She would also like to thank her project editor Angela Baynham and the rest of the creative team at DK; Anita O'Neill, Vicky McIvor, and Professor Barker.

DK Publishing would like to thank Joyce Frye, DO, MBA, FACOG, Research fellow at the Center for Clinical Epidemiology and Biostatistics, University of Pennsylvania for her review of the manuscript; Ann Baggaley for proof-reading; and Sue Bosanko for the index.

NEW PHOTOGRAPHY
Photographer: Caroline Mardon
Photography assistance: Victoria Dawe
Models: Philippa Esson, Elise See Tai, Michelle Horan-Cashmore, Hester Phillips, Jamila Haq, Charmaine Williams, Nicola Bird, Sara Kimmins, Jack Fisher, Abbie and Jake Lawler-Barratt, Raveena Khalsa, Thomas Havelock-Walsh, Taryn Jones, Julie Nicholls, Antonia Nicol, Holly Conroy, Stacy and baby Darcy Free.
DK Publishing would also like to thank the following photography locations: Baring Primary School, The Edgeware Birth Centre, Middlesex and Don't Panic Go Organic food store.

ILLUSTRATIONS
Debbie Maizels and Philip Wilson.

PICTURE CREDITS
DK Publishing would like to thank the following for their kind permission to reproduce their photographs: abbreviations key: r= right; l= left; a= above; b= below; t= top; c= center)
1: Science Photo Library/Ian Hooton; 12: Getty Images/Daniel Bosler; 21: Science Photo Library/Andrew Syred; 22: Getty Images/DTF Productions; 24: Getty Images/Frank Herholdt: 26: Getty Images/Sacha Ajbeszyc; 30: Mediscan/Visuals Unlimited/ Dr David Phillips; 33: Science Photo Library/Dr Yorgos Nikas cl, clb, bl; Eye of Science t; 33: The Wellcome Institute Library, London/Yorgos Nikas br; 35: Science Photo Library/Eye of Science; 37: Science Photo Library/Zephyr; 39: Getty Images/Antonio Mo; 40: Royalty Free Images/Getty; 43: Mother & Baby Picture Library/ Paul Mitchell; 44: Science Photo Library/Dr Najeeb Layyous; 48: Mother & Baby Picture Library/Paul Mitchell; 49: Alamy Images: Andy Bishop; 51: Getty Images/Dennis O'Clair; 52: Prof. J.E. Jirasek MD, DSc; 55: Science Photo Library/Edelmann;

58: Science Photo Library/Edelmann; 59: Mother & Baby Picture Library/Ian Hooton; 60: Getty Images/Ghislain & Marie David de Lossy; 64: Mediscan/ Chineze Otigbah l, r; 68: Science Photo Library/Dr Najeeb Layyous; 71: Rex Features; 74: Getty Images/Chad Ehlers; 75: Courtesy of Bridget Tunnicliffe; 77: Science Photo Library/ Tissuepix; 78: Getty Images/Yoichi Nagata; 82: Science Photo Library/ Genesis Films/ Neil Bromhall; 84: Science Photo Library/GE Medical Systems; 86: Getty Images/Brooke Fasani; 88: Getty Images/Tom Grill; 90: Science Photo Library/GE Medical Systems; 92: Science Photo Library/ Simon Fraser/ Royal Victoria Infirmary, Newcastle Upon Tyne; 106: Science Photo Library/Simon Fraser; 108: Royalty Free Images/Corbis; 111: Mother & Baby Picture Library/ Paul Mitchell; 115: Science Photo Library/Joseph Nettis; 116: Mother & Baby Picture Library/Moose Azim; 118: Mother & Baby Picture Library/ Ruth Jenkinson; 120: Mother & Baby Picture Library/Ruth Jenkinson; 123: Science Photo Library/BSIP, Edwige.

All other images © DK Publishing. For further information see: www.dkimages.com